WALL PILATES WORKOUTS FOR *WOMEN*

Easy-to-Follow & Low-Impact 28-Day Training Program to Feel at Ease in your Body. Tailored Step-by-step Videos and Real Photos to Achieve Balance, Mobility & Power

Thea Morrow

HERE ARE YOUR FREE GIFTS!

SCAN HERE TO GAIN ACCESS

Just point your cellphone's camera at the following QR code and click the link:

YOU WILL GET ACCESS TO:

- **BONUS #1 - Over 100 Step-by-Step Video Tutorials:** Precise video tutorials for each workout, emphasizing safety and correct form, perfect for beginners.

- **BONUS #2 - Ready-to-Print Fitness Planner**: Keep on track with my stylish fitness planner – your ultimate guide to planning workouts, tracking progress, and achieving your fitness goals.

- **BONUS #3 - 7-Day Wall Pilates Training Program for Weight Loss**: An effective, home-based solution for weight reduction. Specifically designed to boost your metabolism and sculpt your body, this digital guide offers concise, equipment-free Wall Pilates workouts designed for quick results. Perfect for anyone who wants to lose weight efficiently without going to the gym.

Introduction

Getting Started with Wall Pilates: A No-Stress Guide to Feeling Great

Welcome to a journey that promises not just to transform your body but to enrich your mind and spirit through the art of Wall Pilates. This book is more than just a collection of exercises; it's a gateway to discovering a stronger, more balanced you. As you turn these pages, you'll embark on an adventure that melds the physical precision of Pilates with the grounding presence of a wall, offering a unique blend of strength, flexibility, and mindfulness.

This guide is designed to be your companion as you navigate this new terrain, with clear, detailed instructions and real-life illustrations that make each pose accessible, regardless of your fitness level.

At the heart of this book lies the conviction that fitness is a holistic journey. We delve into the origins of Wall Pilates, tracing its evolution from a visionary exercise method to its current status as a versatile, home-friendly practice.

Through chapters dedicated to meditation, relaxation, and breathwork, you'll learn how to weave mindfulness into your routine, transforming your practice into a moving meditation that nourishes your soul. The centerpiece of this book, a meticulously crafted 28-day challenge, is designed to gradually build your strength and confidence. Complemented by an exclusive collection of video tutorials, this program offers a comprehensive approach that caters to both beginners and seasoned practitioners. These videos will guide you, step by step, through each movement, ensuring your journey is both safe and deeply rewarding.

Understanding that every woman's journey is unique, you'll find chapters tailored to specific needs—whether you're seeking relief from menstrual discomfort, navigating the physical changes post-pregnancy, or looking for gentle support through menopause.

But perhaps the most crucial message of this book is the importance of staying motivated. Fitness journeys are marathons, not sprints, and this guide is replete with strategies to keep your flame alive.

Embarking on this Wall Pilates journey is about saying yes to a practice that fills you with strength, serenity, and a deep joy. This book is here to hold your hand, cheer you on, and sprinkle a little fun as you discover just how incredible you can feel. So, let's leap into the world of Wall Pilates together – a place where every move is a step closer to a more vibrant, balanced, and joyful you.

Welcome aboard!

Thea Morrow

Starting at the Wall: The Roots and Rise of Wall Pilates

The Origins and Evolution of Wall Pilates

It all began with Joseph Pilates, an innovator far ahead of his time, who believed that mental and physical health were closely connected. He introduced the world to Pilates in the early 20th century, focusing on core strength, flexibility, and mindful movement. But how did we go from classic Pilates to doing planks and stretches against the wall? That's the cool evolution we're diving into.

From Mats to Walls: A Creative Twist

Imagine Joseph Pilates in his studio, surrounded by equipment he designed himself, like the Reformer and the Cadillac. While these machines were fantastic, not everyone had access to them. It was only a matter of time before Pilates enthusiasts and professionals started getting creative. The idea was simple yet revolutionary: use the wall as a tool to enhance Pilates exercises. The wall became a partner in the workout, offering resistance, support, and feedback on alignment and posture. This was a game-changer, especially for those practicing at home or in small spaces. It meant that the core principles of Pilates could be adapted and expanded, making the practice even more accessible and versatile.

Why the Wall?

So, why did the wall become such a central figure in this evolution? It's all about feedback and alignment. When you're doing Pilates against a wall, you immediately know if you're not straight or if one side of your body is doing more work than the other. The wall doesn't lie, and it doesn't let you cheat on your exercises. Plus, it's always there – no special equipment needed, just you and the wall. This evolution wasn't just about practicality; it was about innovation. Pilates has always been a dynamic practice, adapting and growing with each generation. Wall Pilates is a testament to that spirit of innovation, taking the foundational principles Joseph Pilates laid down and pushing them in new directions.

Foundation for Mind and Body: Mindful Movement

Wall Pilates isn't just about where you do it; it's about how you do it and why. It's built on some solid principles that intertwine the mind and body.

First up, we've got mindful movement. This is all about being present and paying attention to each movement you make against that wall. It's not about rushing through the exercises; it's about savoring them, feeling each muscle as it engages, and breathing through every moment. This mindfulness creates a meditative state, turning your workout into a moving meditation. Pretty cool, right?

Core Engagement

The exercises are designed to strengthen your powerhouse, which includes your abs, back, and pelvic muscles. Using the wall helps you engage these muscles more effectively, ensuring that your core gets the love and attention it deserves. This isn't just about getting a toned tummy; it's about building strength that supports your entire body, improving posture, and reducing back pain.

The wall acts like a mirror, giving you instant feedback on your posture and alignment. Leaning, stretching, or pushing against the wall reveals if you're off-center or if you're compensating on one side. This feedback is invaluable, helping you correct your posture not just during your workout, but in everyday life.

Breath Control and Precision

Breath control is another cornerstone of Wall Pilates. The exercises are synced with your breathing, teaching you to inhale and exhale with intention. This controlled breathing enhances your exercises, oxygenates your body, and calms your mind. It's about turning breath into energy that powers your movements, making each session feel like a refreshing breeze.

Wall Pilates is also about precision – doing each movement with purpose and attention to detail. The wall helps you refine your technique, ensuring that every exercise is performed with the utmost care. This focus on precision naturally leads to a flow, a graceful transition from one exercise to the next, making your workout feel like a dance between you and the wall.

Wall Pilates for Pain Relief

Now, let's not forget an essential highlight of Wall Pilates that deserves its own spotlight: pain relief. Whether it's that nagging lower back pain from hours spent at your desk or the shoulder tension that seems to collect the day's stress, Wall Pilates steps in as your personal pain relief therapist.

By focusing on strengthening and stretching, it helps release muscle tension and corrects imbalances that often lead to discomfort. The gentle yet effective support of the wall allows you to safely explore movements that can alleviate pain, making it an ideal practice for those looking to ease their aches without overburdening their bodies.

Essentials for Your Wall Pilates Journey

Embark on your Wall Pilates adventure by finding a wall that speaks to your spirit—a space uncluttered and serene, where your arms can dance freely in the air and your feet can wander a step or two in any direction. Whether it's the cozy corner of your living room, a peaceful spot in your bedroom, or a quiet stretch of hallway, ensure it's a place where freedom and movement harmonize.

The beauty of Wall Pilates lies in its simplicity. Your toolkit just needs: A yoga mat or a soft surface that cradles your body as you move, sit, or lie down. Clothing that feels like a second skin, allowing every stretch and movement to flow unhindered.

Beyond the Wall: Meditation, Relaxation and Breathwork Techniques

Meditation Meets Movement

You might be thinking, "Meditation? But I thought we were here to exercise!" Well, my friend, meditation and Wall Pilates are like peanut butter and jelly – separately great, but together? Magic. Meditation helps you tune into your body, enhancing the mind-body connection that is central to Pilates. It's about bringing a sense of presence and focus to each movement, making your practice not just a workout, but a moving meditation.

Breath as a Bridge

In Wall Pilates, your breath is more than just air moving in and out; it's the bridge that connects your body and mind. As you move through your exercises, let your breath be your guide. Notice the rhythm of your breathing, how it ebbs and flows with your movements, and how it anchors you, keeping you grounded and focused.

As you engage with the wall, whether it's through stretches, strength exercises, or balance work, bring a quality of mindfulness to each movement. Feel the wall against your hands or feet, notice the engagement of your muscles, and observe the sensations in your body without judgment. This mindful awareness transforms each exercise into a moment of meditation, deepening the connection between your physical and mental states.

Ending with Reflection

After your last stretch, take another moment of stillness. Reflect on your practice, acknowledging the work you've done and the space you've created in your body and mind. Ending your session with a few moments of meditation allows you to carry the sense of calm, focus, and connection into the rest of your day.

Pre-Workout Meditation: Setting the Stage

Before you even glance at that wall, let's set the stage for a fantastic session. A pre-workout meditation can help focus your mind, set your intentions, and get you grounded. Here's a simple guide to get you started:

1. **Find Your Spot:** Sit comfortably in front of your wall space, on your mat, with your legs crossed or however you feel best. If sitting on the floor isn't for you, a chair works great too.

2. **Breathe Deep:** Close your eyes and take a few deep breaths. Inhale through your nose, feel your belly rise, and then exhale slowly through your mouth. Let each breath bring you more into the present moment.

3. **Set Your Intention:** Think about what you want to achieve in your session today. Is it strength? Peace? Flexibility? Visualize this intention with each inhale and imagine sending it through your whole body with each exhale.

4. **Visualize Success:** Spend a moment picturing yourself moving through your Wall Pilates routine with ease and grace. Imagine how good you'll feel during and after the workout.

5. **Gently Begin:** Open your eyes when you're ready, feeling focused and prepared to tackle your workout with all you've got.

Post-Workout Meditation: Soaking in the Goodness

After you've stretched, strengthened, and sweat it out, a post-workout meditation can help you absorb all the benefits of your practice, leaving you feeling refreshed and rejuvenated. Here's how to wrap up your session:

1. **Cool Down First:** After your last exercise, take a few minutes for some gentle stretching or simply lying down in a comfortable position, letting your body start to relax.

2. **Reflect on Gratitude:** Close your eyes and focus on your breath again. This time, think about what you're grateful for from your session – maybe it's your body's strength, a moment of clarity, or simply the time you dedicated to yourself.

3. **Scan Your Body:** Mentally scan your body from head to toe, noticing any areas of new openness or energy. Acknowledge the work you've done and thank your body for all its hard work.

4. **Carry Forward the Calm:** Visualize the calm, strength, and balance you've cultivated during your practice extending beyond your workout, into the rest of your day or evening.

5. **Return Gently:** When you're ready, gently open your eyes, bringing the sense of peace and accomplishment with you as you move forward.

Incorporating these guided meditations before and after your Wall Pilates workouts can profoundly impact your practice, transforming it into a more holistic experience. They help bridge the gap between physical exercise and mental well-being, ensuring you not only look great but feel fantastic too.

Visualization: Your Relaxation Superpower

Visualization, or guided imagery, can transport you from your workout space to a place of profound peace and relaxation. Here's how to harness this superpower:

1. **Get Comfy:** After your workout, find a comfortable position, either sitting or lying down.

2. **Picture Peace:** Close your eyes and imagine a place that represents ultimate relaxation to you. It could be a beach, a mountain retreat, or a cozy nook in your home.

3. **Engage Your Senses:** In your mind's eye, explore this place using all your senses. What do you see? What can you hear? Is there a scent in the air? The more vivid, the better.

4. **Breathe in Calm:** With each inhale, draw in the peace and tranquility of this place. With each exhale, release any remaining tension from your body.

Understanding Breath and Its Impact on Well-being

Our breath is the bridge between our body and mind, directly influencing our stress levels, mood, and even our body's ability to heal and perform. When we breathe deeply and intentionally, we signal to our nervous system that it's time to relax, moving away from the fight-or-flight response and into a state of calm and restoration.

Deep, mindful breathing increases oxygen flow, boosts energy levels, and helps clear the mind. It's like hitting the reset button on your stress levels, making it easier to tackle challenges with a sense of calm and clarity. In the context of Wall Pilates, understanding this powerful connection between breath and well-being sets the foundation for a practice that not only strengthens your body but also nurtures your soul.

Breath Techniques for Energy and Relaxation

Now, let's dive into some breath techniques that you can use to supercharge your Wall Pilates practice, whether you need a boost of energy, a moment of relaxation, or a sharper focus.

Energizing Breath: The 3-Part Breath

*   Start by standing or sitting tall, with your back gently touching the wall for alignment.

*   Inhale deeply through your nose, filling your abdomen, then your chest, and finally letting the breath rise into your upper chest and collarbones.

*   Exhale smoothly through your nose, releasing the air from your upper chest, chest, and then abdomen.

*   Repeat for 3-5 cycles when you need an energy boost before or during your workout.

Relaxing Breath: The 4-7-8 Technique

*   Sit or lie down comfortably, using the wall as support for your back if sitting.

*   Inhale quietly through your nose for 4 seconds.

*   Hold your breath for 7 seconds.

*   Exhale completely through your mouth, making a whoosh sound, for 8 seconds.

*   Repeat the cycle four times to help you relax after your workout or to calm your mind before starting.

Mindful Breathing: The Anchor of Relaxation

Mindful breathing is a simple yet powerful tool you can use anytime, anywhere, to center and calm yourself. Post-Wall Pilates, it's like a cool-down for your mind. Try this:

1. **Find Your Breath:** Sit or lie down and place one hand on your chest, the other on your belly.

2. **Inhale Slowly:** Inhale slowly through your nose, feeling your belly rise, then your chest.

3. **Exhale Completely:** Exhale through your mouth, letting your chest fall, then your belly, pushing all the air out.

4. **Repeat and Focus:** Continue for several minutes, focusing solely on your breath. If your mind wanders, gently bring it back to your breathing.

Integrating Breathwork with Wall Pilates Movements

Breath isn't just a background player in Wall Pilates; it's part of the main act. Integrating breathwork with your movements enhances the effectiveness of each exercise, deepens your connection to your body, and turns your practice into a rhythmic dance between movement and breath.

- **Coordinate Your Movements:** In general, inhale to prepare or extend, and exhale to engage or contract. For example, inhale as you lengthen your spine against the wall, and exhale as you engage your core in a wall sit.

- **Use Breath as a Guide:** Let your breath lead your movements, not the other way around. This ensures you're moving mindfully and maintaining a pace that keeps your practice flowing and focused.

- **Mindful Transitions:** Pay attention to your breath even between exercises. Use these moments to reconnect with your intention, check in with your body, and prepare your mind for the next movement.

By mastering breathwork in Wall Pilates, you unlock a powerful tool for enhancing every aspect of your practice. From energizing your body and calming your mind, breath is your constant companion on the journey to a stronger, more balanced you.

Wall Pilates Techniques and Exercises: An Overview

Within these chapters, you'll find a diverse array of exercises categorized by their primary focus areas: **Warm-Up and Cool-Down, Core Strengthening and Stability, Lower Body Power, Upper Body Strength**. Each exercise has been carefully selected and described to ensure you can practice safely, effectively, and with confidence right from your home and without any equipment besides a mat.

To help you navigate through the exercises and tailor your practice to your current fitness level, I have employed a simple yet effective ranking system. Here's a quick breakdown:

- **Rank 1 (Beginner):** These exercises are your building blocks. They're designed to introduce you to the fundamentals of Wall Pilates, focusing on basic movements that require minimal muscle engagement and physical demand. Perfect for those new to Pilates or looking for gentle exercise options.

- **Rank 2 (Intermediate):** As you grow more comfortable with the basics, these exercises will challenge you a bit more, incorporating moderate complexity and muscle engagement. Ideal for practitioners ready to take their workout up a notch.

- **Rank 3 (Advanced):** These exercises demand a higher level of skill, strength, and balance. They offer a challenge to those looking to push their limits and explore the full potential of Wall Pilates.

The Importance of Warm-Up & Cool-Down Exercises

In my Wall Pilates journey, I've discovered the power of beginning each session with warm-up exercises. These aren't mere movements; they're a transition from stillness to activity, a warm invitation to my body and mind. Through these initial stretches, my heart rate gently rises, my muscles receive a fresh supply of blood, and my joints prepare for the day's workout. It's a time not just for physical readiness but for focusing my mind on the breaths and movements ahead.

The importance of cooling down mirrors that of warming up, grounding me after my practice. It's a gentle return to daily life, letting my heart rate slow and my muscles relax and stretch. More than a recovery phase, it's a moment to appreciate my body's effort, staving off next-day soreness and grounding me in gratitude for the work accomplished.

Core Strengthening and Stability

At the heart of Wall Pilates, and indeed at the center of my practice, lies core strengthening and stability. It's fascinating to realize that the 'core' encompasses far more than the abdominal muscles; it includes the back, hips, and pelvic muscles, forming the very essence of physical health. A strong core for me means more than an aesthetic silhouette; it's about enhancing my posture, safeguarding against injuries, and improving my overall performance in every physical endeavor I undertake.

Upper Body Strength and Flexibility

When I turn my attention to upper body exercises within my Wall Pilates routine, I'm reminded of their significance beyond just achieving a harmonious physique. These exercises empower me to tackle daily tasks effortlessly, uphold a healthy posture, and safeguard myself from potential injuries. Through a series of carefully selected movements, I work towards not only strengthening but also increasing the flexibility of my shoulders, arms, chest, and back, ensuring a well-rounded approach to fitness.

Lower Body Fortitude for Sculpting Stability and Grace

And let's not overlook the foundation of it all—the lower body. It's the source of our strength and stability, supporting everything from our posture to our mobility. In this book, I delve into exercises aimed at sculpting the legs, boosting glute strength, and enhancing overall stability. It's a journey towards not just an aesthetically pleasing lower body, but one brimming with health, capable of carrying me through life's daily activities with ease and grace.

Unlocking More: 100+ Exclusive Wall Pilates Videos

Beyond the extensive insights and the transformative 28-Day Challenge in my book, I'm excited to offer you an exclusive opportunity to deepen your Wall Pilates journey. By becoming part of my community, you gain FREE access to an extensive collection of over 100 premium Wall Pilates video tutorials.

These videos enrich the book's content, serving as a dynamic _visual companion_ to demonstrate each exercise with clarity and detail. Ideal for visual learners or those fine-tuning their technique, this resource ensures you practice with both confidence and precision. Notably, my expansive video series doesn't just revisit the foundational exercises outlined in the 28-Day Challenge; it expands into additional routines focused on addressing women's specific health concerns.

In writing my book on wall Pilates, I faced a significant decision regarding the use of imagery. Initially, the idea of colorful images to illustrate the exercises was tempting. However, I quickly realized that color printing with 200 + images significantly increases production costs, which could have necessitated compromises in other areas. I wanted my book to be as comprehensive and accessible as possible, filled with a rich array of content and workouts to benefit readers at every stage of their fitness journey. Thus, I chose to use black and white images. As a result, readers now have access to twice as many exercises and in-depth discussions than they might find in similar, color-illustrated books.

This decision not only helped manage the printing costs but also allowed me to include more exercises and detailed instructions, making the book richer in content. I complemented the book with an online video library to ensure that if any workout is not clear enough through the black and white images, a visual, dynamic representation is just a click away. This hybrid approach—combining the depth of a printed book with the clarity of video demonstrations—reflects my commitment to providing valuable, accessible guidance to my readers.

28 Days to a New You: The 28-Day Wall Pilates Challenge

I'm excited to present a special feature of my book – the 28-Day Challenge Program. This program is thoughtfully designed with beginners in mind, focusing on low-impact exercises that are gentle on the body yet incredibly effective in building strength, enhancing flexibility, and improving overall well-being.

Structure of the Program

The challenge is structured as a **7-Day routine** that you'll **repeat over four consecutive weeks**, making up a comprehensive _28-Day Training Program_. Each day features a series of **10 meticulously chosen** exercises. You're encouraged to perform each exercise for **1 minute**, ensuring that collectively, they comprise a balanced **10-minute daily workout routine**:

- **1 Warm-Up Exercise**: Start each session with a warm-up exercise to gently prepare your body and mind for the workout ahead. This initial step increases blood flow, enhances flexibility, and reduces the risk of injury, setting a positive tone for your practice.

- **2 Core Exercises**: Strengthen and stabilize your powerhouse with two core-focused exercises. These movements are essential for building a strong foundation, improving posture, and supporting overall body function.

- **4 Lower Body Exercises**: The bulk of your daily routine concentrates on the lower body—your legs, glutes, and hips. These exercises are designed to build strength, enhance flexibility, and improve balance, providing a solid foundation for your body.

- **2 Upper Body Exercises**: Tone and fortify your upper body, including shoulders, arms, and chest, with two targeted exercises. Building upper body strength is crucial for daily activities and complements your core and lower body work.

- **1 Cool-Down Exercise**: Conclude each session with a cool-down exercise to relax and stretch your muscles, helping to prevent soreness and promote recovery. This final step also offers a moment of reflection and gratitude for your body's efforts.

Integrating Meditation and Breathwork into Your Daily Routine

Inside the chapter " Beyond the Wall: Meditation, Relaxation and Breathwork Techniques, "we explored the essential role these practices play at every stage of your routine. Before exercises, they set a foundation of focus and calm, preparing both mind and body. During your workout, breathwork enhances each movement's effectiveness, fostering a deeper connection and mindfulness.

Afterward, meditation aids in relaxation and recovery, consolidating the physical and mental benefits of your session. I encourage you to incorporate these practices whenever you feel the need. Whether you're seeking mental clarity before starting your day or looking to enhance your focus during your routine.

28-Day Wall Pilates Challenge

Days	Warm Up	Core	Lower Body	Upper Body	Cool Down
1,8 15,22	Alternating Wall Circles	Seated Thoracic Rotations, Wall Crunch	Wall Side to Side Lunges, Wall Sit, Wall Curtsy Lunges, Sumo Squats	Wall Shoulder Taps, Wall Push Ups	Windshield Wipers
2,9 16,23	Wall Calf Stretch	Wall Reach Through Crunch, Wall Cross body Crunches	Wall Sit with Leg Extension, Wall Sit Clamshells, Wall Squats, Wall Clamshells	Wall Thread the Needle, Wall Cobra Push Up	Wall Frog Stretch
3,10 17,24	Wall Quad Stretch	Wall Assisted Plank, Wall Mountain Climbers	Standing Hip Abduction, Wall Plié Squat with Heel Lifts, Wall Plié Squat Pulses, Wall Sit with Heel Lifts	Wall Kneeling Child's Pose, Wall Kneeling Push Up	Standing Forward Fold
4,11 18,25	Thoracic Rotations	Wall Cross Body Mountain Climbers, Wall Elevated Plank	Wall Glute Bridges, Wall Glute Bridges Clamshells, Wall Single Leg Glute Bridge, Wall Side Lunges	Wall Single Arm Triceps Press, Wall Diamond Push Up	Wall Standing Child's Pose
5,12 19,26	Wall Chest Stretch	Plank Wall Taps, Wall Cross body Toe Touches Crunches	Wall Marching Glute Bridge, Wall Walking Glute Bridge, Wall Glute Kickbacks, Wall Elevated Split Squat	Wall Arm Angels, Wall Arm Butterflies	Wall Reclined Pigeon
6,13 20,27	Wall hip Flexor Stretch	Wall Elevated Plank Side Steps, Wall Standing Knee Drives	Wall Glute Kickbacks Pulses, Wall Glute Rainbow, Hip Adduction, Single Leg Bridge Leg Circles	Wall Triceps Press, Wall Side Bends	Hamstring Stretch
7,14 21,28	Standing Wall Hip Circles	Wall Pilates 100's, Double Leg Stretch	Wall Reverse Lunges, Wall Diamonds, Glute Bridge Pulses, Wall Laying Hip Adductions	Wall Commando Planks, Wall pike	Leg swings

Days 1-8-15-22: Embarking on Your 28-Day Wall Pilates Transformation

Welcome to the start of your Wall Pilates journey! Today marks the beginning of a 28-Day Training Program designed to guide you towards greater mobility, strength, and overall well-being, all within the convenience of your home.

Our focus today is on introducing you to foundational movements that warm you up, target crucial muscle groups, and wrap up with a relaxing cool-down, ensuring a comprehensive workout experience. Let's explore the lineup for today's session:

Warm-Up: Alternating Wall Circles

Kickstart your routine with *Alternating Wall Circles*, a gentle exercise to mobilize your shoulders and upper back. This movement prepares your body for the workout ahead, promoting flexibility and proper posture, setting the tone for a productive session.

Core: Seated Thoracic Rotations & Wall Crunch

Shift focus to your core with *Seated Thoracic Rotations*, aimed at loosening your spine and improving mid-back mobility. This prepares you for a stronger and more effective core workout.

Continue strengthening your core with *Wall Crunches*, a unique variation of the traditional crunch that challenges your abdominal muscles by incorporating wall resistance. This exercise is crucial for enhancing core stability, which supports your overall fitness and daily movements.

Lower Body: Wall Side to Side Lunges, Wall Sit, Wall Curtsy Lunges, Sumo Squats

Dive into lower body work starting with *Wall Side to Side Lunges*, engaging your thighs and glutes and improving lateral mobility. Follow up with the *Wall Sit* for endurance and strength, focusing on your quadriceps.

Incorporate *Wall Curtsy Lunges* to target your glutes and thighs, emphasizing balance and coordination. Finish the lower body segment with *Sumo Squats*, focusing on the inner thighs and glutes to promote strength and flexibility.

Upper Body: Wall Shoulder Taps, Wall Push Ups

For upper body strength, begin with *Wall Shoulder Taps*, which improve shoulder stability and core engagement. Follow with *Wall Push Ups* to build strength in your chest, shoulders, and triceps, enhancing muscle tone and endurance.

Cool-Down: Windshield Wipers

Conclude your workout with *Windshield Wipers*, focusing on relaxing your lower back and hips, reducing tension, and improving flexibility in the lumbar region, leaving you refreshed and rejuvenated.

Each of the 10 exercises should be performed for **1 minute**, amounting to a total of **10 minutes of focused, effective Wall Pilates work**. This time-efficient routine is designed to fit seamlessly into your day, ensuring you can maintain consistency and enjoy the transformative benefits of Wall Pilates.

Alternating Wall Circles

28-Day Challenge
Days 1-8-15-22

BENEFITS

- Enhances shoulder mobility and flexibility.
- Engages core muscles for stability during rotation.
- Improves coordination and opens the chest.

TIPS

- Keep the core engaged to stabilize your posture during the circles.
- Focus on full, controlled circles to maximize shoulder mobility.
- Ensure both feet are firmly planted to maintain balance.
- Alternate arms smoothly for balanced shoulder activation.
- Common Mistakes: Moving too quickly can reduce the effectiveness of the stretch, and not completing the full circle may limit mobility benefits.

1

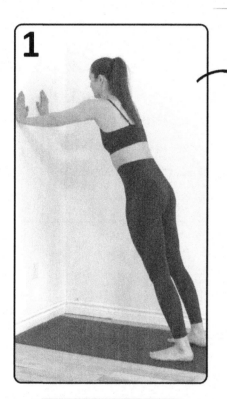

Stand with your feet shoulder-width apart facing the wall. Extend your arms out, placing your hands onto the wall.

2

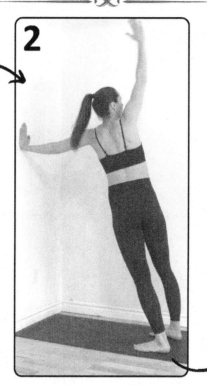

Take a step back with both feet. Lift and rotate one of your arms backwards, opening your body up to that side.

3

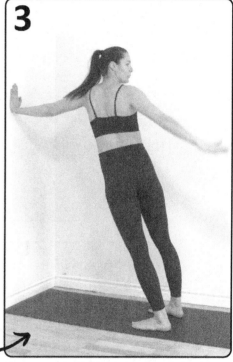

Once your arm is back in its starting position, repeat on the other side.

Seated Thoracic Rotations

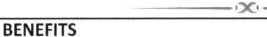

BENEFITS

- Mobilizes and stretches the thoracic spine.
- Encourages rotational flexibility and core engagement.
- Can alleviate mid-back stiffness and improve posture.

TIPS

- Sit with knees bent and lean slightly back to engage the core.
- Keep movements smooth as you rotate and reach to touch the floor. Use your core muscles to control the rotation and support your spine.
- Alternate sides evenly to promote balanced mobility.
- Common Mistakes: Rotating too quickly or not engaging the core can reduce effectiveness and risk discomfort.

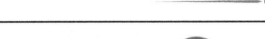

1

> Start seated with your knees bent at a 45-degree angle and your toes on the wall. Keep your knees slightly bent, and lean a bit backward. Place your hands together in front of you.

> From here, open your arm and body to one side, and touch the floor behind you.

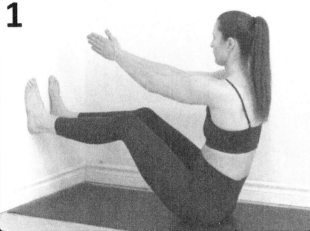

2

3

> Return to the starting position (1) and repeat on the other side.

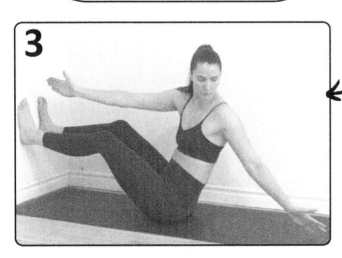

Wall Crunch

BENEFITS

- Strengthens the abdominal muscles, particularly the rectus abdominis.
- Enhances core stability and supports better posture.
- Prepares the body for more advanced abdominal exercises.

TIPS

- Place your feet flat against the wall with knees bent to ensure proper alignment. Keep your movements slow and controlled, focusing on engaging your core.
- Avoid pulling on your neck with your hands.
- Exhale as you lift up to deepen the abdominal contraction.
- Common Mistakes: Twisting the neck or using momentum instead of controlled abdominal engagement can reduce effectiveness and risk neck strain.

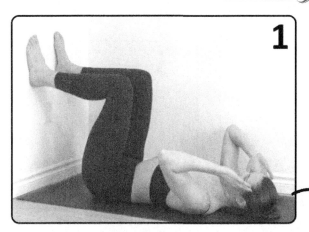

1

Lie flat on your back with your feet on the wall and your knees bent at a 90-degree angle.

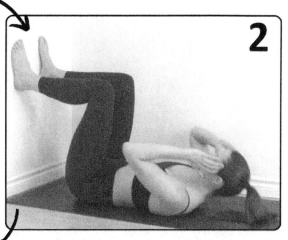

2

Bend your elbows and place your hands by the sides of your head.

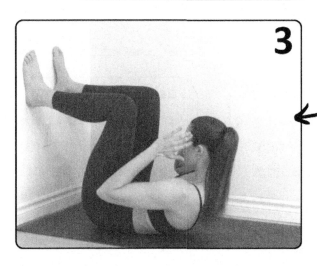

3

Contract your abdominals to lift your shoulder blades off the ground. Slowly lower yourself back down in a controlled manner and repeat.

Wall Side to Side Lunges

BENEFITS

- Improves lower body strength, focusing on the glutes, thighs, and hips.
- Enhances flexibility and range of motion in the hips and inner thighs.
- Promotes balance and stability through dynamic movement.

TIPS

- Use the wall for balance, allowing you to focus on the depth and form of your lunge. Keep the heel of the bent knee grounded to engage the muscles effectively. Push your hips back as you lunge to maintain alignment and protect your knees.
- Ensure a controlled movement, aiming for a smooth transition between sides.
- Common Mistakes: Leaning too far forward can strain the back, and not bending the knee to 90 degrees may reduce the effectiveness of the lunge.

1

2

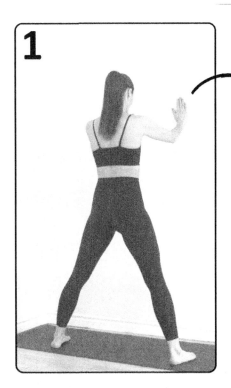

3

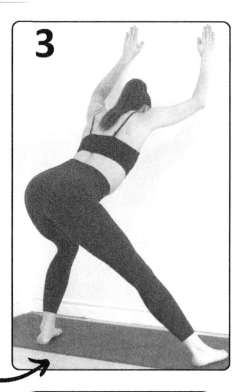

Stand facing the wall with your feet in a wide stance. Place your hands on the wall for support.

Hinge your hips back and bend your knee to a 90-degree angle towards one side.

Push through the heel of your bent knee to come back up and mirror the movement on the other side.

Wall Sit

BENEFITS

- Strengthens the quadriceps, glutes, and hamstrings.
- Improves lower body endurance and stability.
- Enhances core strength and posture.

TIPS

- Ensure your back is flat against the wall throughout the exercise.
- Keep knees aligned over ankles, not extending past the toes.
- Engage your core to support your back and enhance stability.
- Focus on breathing evenly to maintain the position comfortably.
- Common Mistakes: Dropping the hips below knee level can strain the knees, and losing contact with the wall may decrease the effectiveness of the exercise.

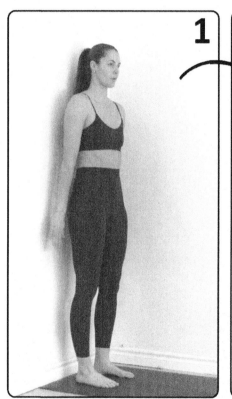 **1**

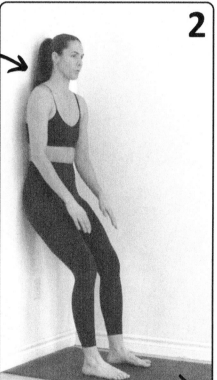 **2**

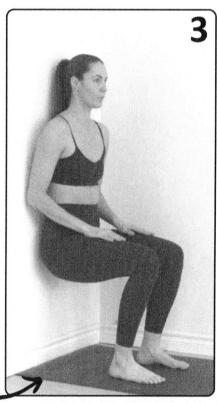 **3**

Stand with your back against a wall and your feet hip-width apart, slightly away from the wall.

Squat down until your knees are bent at a 90-degree angle.Keep your back straight against the wall and your knees directly above your ankles. Hold this seated position. Slowly push through your heels to stand back up once completed.

Wall Curtsy Lunges

BENEFITS

- Targets and tones the glutes, particularly the gluteus medius for a rounded shape.
- Strengthens the thighs and hip stability.
- Enhances coordination and balance with the cross-body movement pattern.

TIPS

- Use the wall for balance, keeping the pressure light to focus on leg work.
- Ensure the back knee lowers directly towards the floor, maintaining the curtsy posture.
- Keep your chest lifted and core engaged to support your upper body.
- Push through the front heel to return to standing, maximizing glute engagement.
- Common Mistakes: Losing posture or balance during the movement reduces effectiveness.

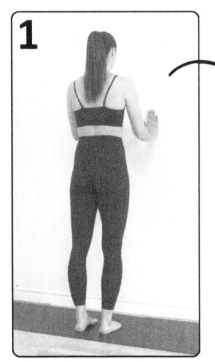
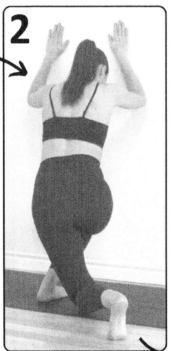
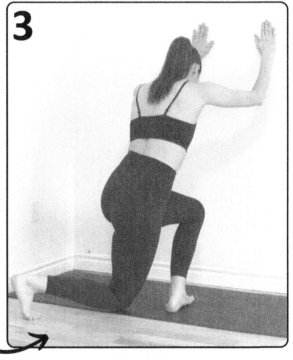

Stand facing a wall, feet hip-width apart. Place your hands on the wall at about chest height for support.

Step back and behind your right leg with your left foot, creating a curtsy-like position. Lower your body into a lunge with both knees at 90-degree angles. Push through your right heel to return to the starting position (1) and repeat on the other side. Continue alternating between your right and left leg.

Wall Sumo Squats

BENEFITS

- Targets the glutes, inner thighs, and quadriceps.
- Enhances hip flexibility and strengthens the lower body.
- Improves posture and lower body alignment.

TIPS

- Keep your feet wide and toes pointed outward to engage the target muscles effectively.
- Ensure your knees track over your toes and avoid letting them collapse inward.
- Push through your heels to return to the starting position, engaging your glutes and inner thighs.
- Maintain a straight back and engaged core throughout the movement.
- Common Mistakes: Not squatting deep enough can reduce the effectiveness of the exercise.

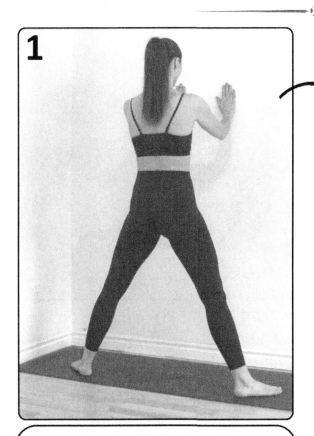

1

Stand facing the wall with your feet in a wide stance and your feet externally rotated. Place your hands on the wall.

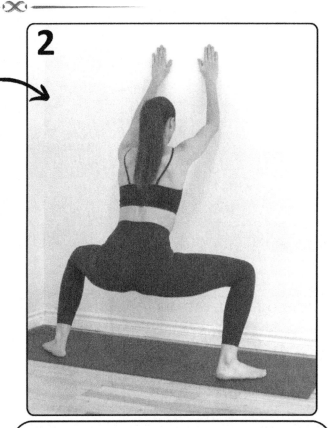

2

Squat down until your knees are at a 90-degree angle and your thighs are parallel to the ground. Push through your heels to come back up and repeat.

Wall Shoulder Taps

BENEFITS

- Enhances core stability and strength.
- Improves balance and coordination.
- Engages shoulder and arm muscles.

TIPS

- Maintain a strong, straight body line. Move hands slowly and with control. Keep hips steady, avoid rocking. Maintain a strong core throughout to stabilize your body. Keep your hips level to avoid rocking side to side.
- Focus on controlled movements for maximum effectiveness.
- Common Mistakes: Letting the lower back sag and overreaching can disrupt form and balance.

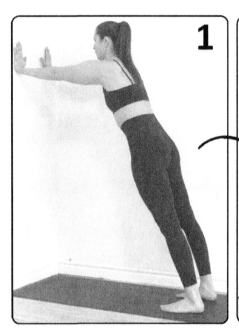

1

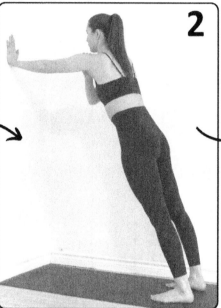

2

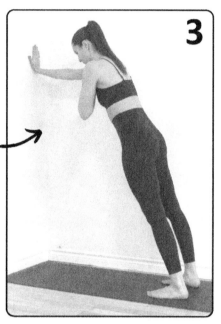

3

Stand facing the wall with your feet hip-width apart. Place your hands on the wall at shoulder level. Step both feet back one step. Hold this wall plank position.

Slowly lift your right hand off the wall and tap your left shoulder.

Place it back on the wall and repeat on the other side. Continue, alternating sides each time.

BENEFITS

- Builds strength in chest, shoulders, and triceps.
- Engages and strengthens the core.
- Improves posture and upper body stability.

TIPS

- Keep feet hip-width for balance; adjust distance for comfort.
- Engage your core throughout to protect your back.
- Lower with control; focus on smooth movements.
- Ensure full extension during the push to maximize benefits.
- Common Mistakes: Arching the back or not moving through the full range can diminish effectiveness and risk strain.

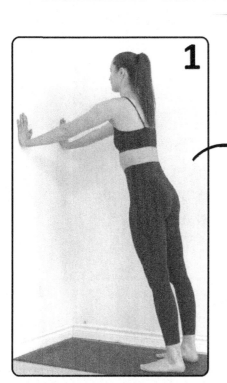

1

Stand facing the wall with your feet hip-width apart. Place your hands on the wall at shoulder level. Step your feet back one step. Hold this position by keeping your core engaged and back straight.

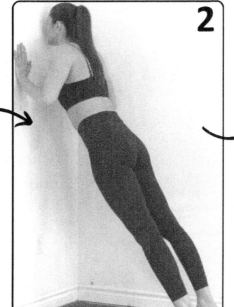

2

Bend your elbows and lower yourself to bring your chest towards the wall.

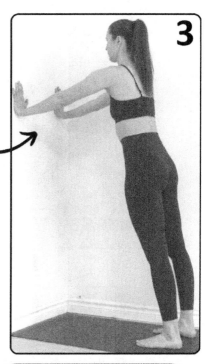

3

Push through the palms of your hands to come back up and repeat.

Windshield Wipers

BENEFITS

- Enhances core strength and oblique activation.
- Improves lower back and hip flexibility.
- Promotes spinal mobility and stability.

TIPS

- Keep arms extended and pressed to the ground for stability.
- Move knees side to side with control.
- Aim to keep both shoulders in contact with the ground to ensure a proper twist.
- Breathe smoothly throughout the movement, coordinating with each side switch.
- Common Mistakes: Lifting the shoulders off the ground can reduce the effectiveness of the spinal twist, and moving the knees too quickly may not engage the core fully.

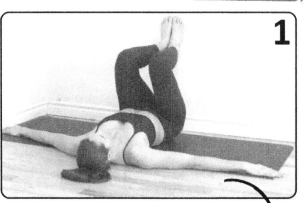

1

Lie on your back with your knees and feet together up on the wall. Keep your knees bent at a 90-degree angle. Extend your arms to the side.

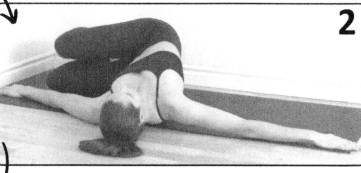

2

From here, bring your knees towards the floor to your left side.

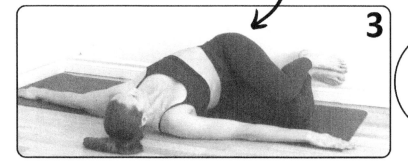

3

Bring them up, and do the same thing on your right side

Days 2-9-16-23: Continuing Your Wall Pilates Journey

Welcome to Day 2 of your transformative 28-day Wall Pilates challenge. Building on the foundation laid on Day 1, today's routine will introduce new exercises to further engage your muscles, enhance your flexibility, and continue to foster a deep connection between your mind and body. Let's dive into today's detailed workout plan:

Warm-Up: Wall Calf Stretch

Ease into today's session with the _Wall Calf Stretch_, aiming to loosen your calf muscles and Achilles tendon. This vital warm-up prepares your lower body for the exercises ahead, promoting mobility and preventing injuries.

Core: Wall Reach Through Crunch & Wall Cross body Crunches

Strengthen your core further with the _Wall Reach Through Crunch_, focusing on engaging your deep abdominal muscles and enhancing coordination.

Continue with _Wall Cross body Crunches_ to target your obliques, promoting core stability and improving your torso's rotational movement. These core exercises are fundamental for a strong foundation, supporting overall movement and stability.

Lower Body: Wall Sit with Leg Extension, Wall Sit Clamshells, Wall Squats, Wall Clamshells

Intensify your lower body workout with _Wall Sit with Leg Extension_, challenging your endurance and strengthening your quads through controlled leg movements.

Add variation with _Wall Sit Clamshells_ to engage your glutes and outer thighs, promoting hip stability.

Wall Squats will further build your lower body strength, focusing on your glutes, thighs, and calves with a functional movement that enhances everyday mobility.

Incorporate _Wall Clamshells_ as a focused exercise to target the glutes and hips, improving lateral stability and strength.

Upper Body: Wall Thread the Needle, Wall Cobra Push Up

Open up your upper body with _Wall Thread the Needle_, a dynamic stretch that releases tension in your shoulders and upper back, enhancing flexibility.

Strengthen your upper body with _Wall Cobra Push Ups_, focusing on your chest, triceps, and shoulders. This exercise also encourages back extension, contributing to a balanced upper body workout.

Cool-Down: Wall Frog Stretch

Conclude your routine with the _Wall Frog Stretch_, a gentle yet effective way to relax your hips, groin, and inner thighs. This cool-down exercise ensures you finish your session feeling stretched, relaxed, and rejuvenated. Each exercise should be performed for **1 minute**, culminating in a **10-minute total workout** that continues to build upon your Pilates foundation.

Wall Calf Stretch - Left

BENEFITS

- Stretches and relieves tightness in the calf muscles.
- Enhances flexibility and mobility in the lower legs.
- Can help prevent calf muscle injuries and aid in recovery post-activity.

TIPS

- Keep the heel of the stretching leg firmly on the ground to maximize the calf stretch.
- Lean into the wall only as much as needed to feel a comfortable stretch, without straining.
- Use controlled movements to enter and exit the stretch, maintaining steady breathing.
- Perform the stretch on both sides to ensure balanced flexibility.
- Common Mistakes: Not keeping the heel down or overstretching can lead to reduced effectiveness or potential strain.

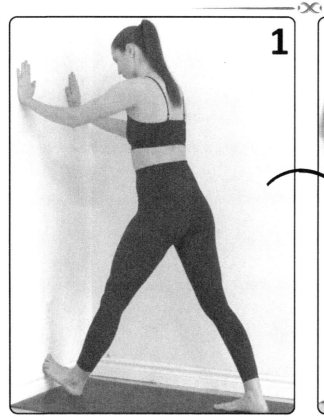

1

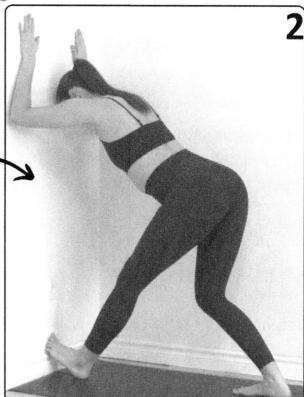

2

Stand with your feet hip-width apart facing the wall, an arm's length away. Extend your arm out to shoulder height and place your palms on the wall. Put your left toes on the wall while keeping your left heel on the floor.

From this position, lean your torso and head towards the wall, feeling a stretch in your calf. Come back up and repeat for the duration of this exercise

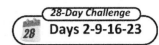
BENEFITS

- Stretches and relieves tightness in the calf muscles.
- Enhances flexibility and mobility in the lower legs.
- Can help prevent calf muscle injuries and aid in recovery post-activity.

TIPS

- Keep the heel of the stretching leg firmly on the ground to maximize the calf stretch.
- Lean into the wall only as much as needed to feel a comfortable stretch, without straining.
- Use controlled movements to enter and exit the stretch, maintaining steady breathing.
- Perform the stretch on both sides to ensure balanced flexibility.
- Common Mistakes: Not keeping the heel down or overstretching can lead to reduced effectiveness or potential strain.

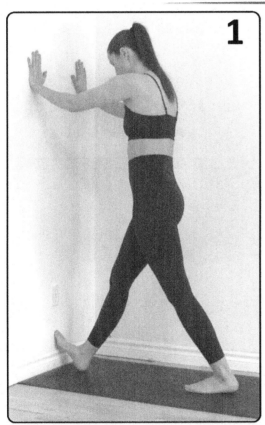

1

Stand with your feet hip-width apart facing the wall, an arm's length away. Extend your arm out to shoulder height and place your palms on the wall. Put your right toes on the wall while keeping your right heel on the floor.

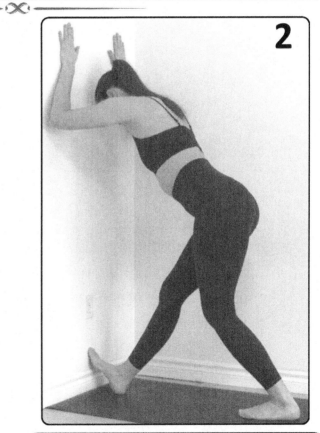

2

From this position, lean your torso and head towards the wall, feeling a stretch in your calf. Come back up and repeat for the duration of this exercise

Wall Reach Through Crunch

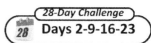

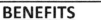

BENEFITS

- Targets the deep core muscles, enhancing abdominal strength.
- Improves the rectus abdominis
- Increases core control and stability.

TIPS

- Keep your feet pressed against the wall to maintain a stable base.
- Engage your core as you reach through, focusing on a full contraction. Move your arms and shoulders, not your neck, to reach through your knees.
- Inhale as you prepare and exhale during the reach to maximize core engagement.
- Common Mistakes: Avoid using momentum or arching the lower back, which can lead to strain and diminish the exercise's effectiveness.

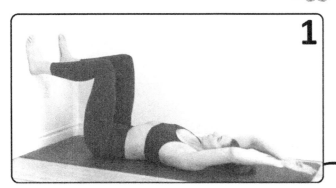

1

Lie flat on your back with your feet on the wall and your knees bent at a 90-degree angle. Extend your arms over your head and put your hands together.

2

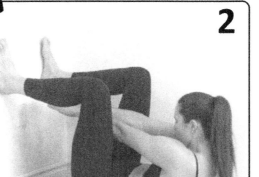

Contract your abdominals and bring your hands between your knees, as far as you can reach.

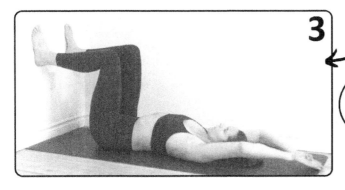

3

Slowly lower yourself back to the starting position and repeat.

Wall Cross Body Crunches

 28-Day Challenge Days 2-9-16-23

BENEFITS

- Specifically targets and strengthens the obliques for improved waist definition.
- Enhances core stability and rotational mobility.
- Supports functional movements and balance in daily activities.

TIPS

- Ensure your feet remain flat against the wall for stability.
- Focus on rotating your torso, not just moving your elbow, to engage the obliques fully. Alternate sides smoothly, maintaining even reps on each side for balance.
- Keep the movement controlled, using your core muscles to lift and twist.
- Common Mistakes: Pulling on the neck or losing contact with the wall can reduce the effectiveness and risk discomfort.

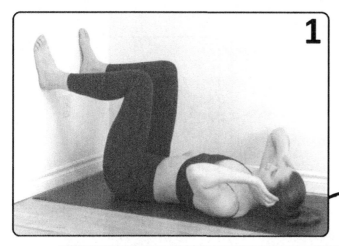

1 Lie flat on your back with your feet on the wall and your knees bent at a 90-degree angle. Bend your elbows and bring your hands to the sides of your head.

Contract your abdominals to lift your shoulder blades off the ground. Reach your right elbow towards your left knee.

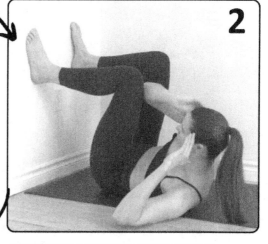

2

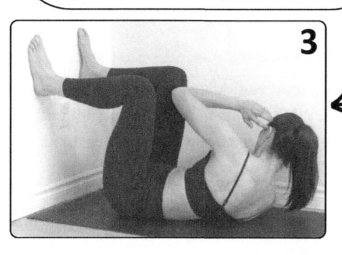

3

Slowly lower yourself back down and repeat, this time reaching your left elbow towards your right knee.

Wall Sit with Leg Extension

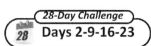
28-Day Challenge
Days 2-9-16-23

BENEFITS

- Strengthens the quadriceps, glutes, and hamstrings.
- Enhances lower body endurance and stability.
- Improves balance and core engagement.

TIPS

- Ensure your back remains flat against the wall throughout the exercise.
- Keep the non-lifting leg stable and bent at a 90-degree angle.
- Extend one leg at a time smoothly, focusing on engaging the quadriceps.
- Alternate legs without compromising your seated wall sit posture.
- Common Mistakes: Allowing the back to come off the wall or the seated knee to move forward past the ankles can reduce effectiveness and risk injury.

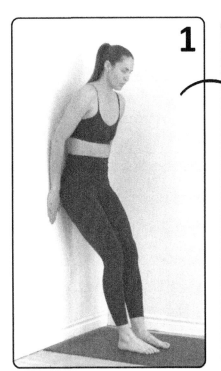
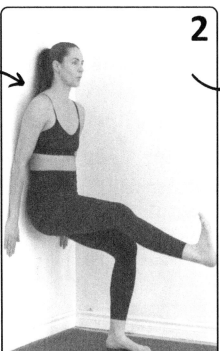
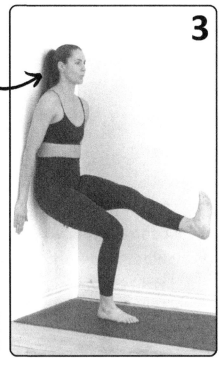

Stand with your back against a wall and your feet hip-width apart, slightly away from the wall.

Squat down until your knees are bent at a 90-degree angle. While sitting in this position, lift and extend one of your legs by contracting your quad. Alternate between the legs.

Wall Sit Clamshells

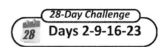
BENEFITS

- Targets and strengthens the glutes, particularly the gluteus medius.
- Enhances hip stability and mobility.
- Improves lower body endurance and control.

TIPS

- Maintain a deep wall sit position to keep the focus on the lower body. Open your knees as wide as comfortably possible, focusing on engaging the glutes.
- Control the movement both outward and inward to maximize muscle engagement.
- Common Mistakes: Allowing the hips to rise or the lower back to arch can diminish the effectiveness of the exercise and potentially strain the back.

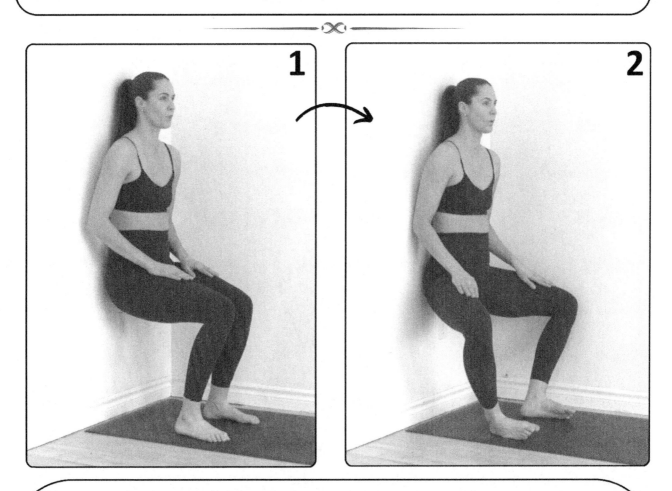

Stand with your back against a wall and your feet hip-width apart, slightly away from the wall. Squat down until your knees are bent at a 90-degree angle. Open your knees out to the side, contracting your glutes at the top of this movement. Bring your knees back (1) in and repeat.

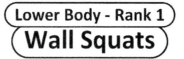

Lower Body - Rank 1
Wall Squats

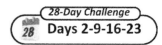

28-Day Challenge
Days 2-9-16-23

BENEFITS

- Strengthens the quadriceps, hamstrings, and glutes.
- Improves lower body stability and endurance.
- Enhances knee and hip mobility.

TIPS

- Keep your back flat against the wall throughout the movement.
- Ensure your knees do not extend past your toes when squatting down.
- Push through your heels to return to the starting position, focusing on activating your glutes. Maintain a controlled pace, focusing on the quality of movement over speed.
- Common Mistakes: Rushing the squat or allowing the knees to cave inward can lead to less effective muscle engagement and potential strain.

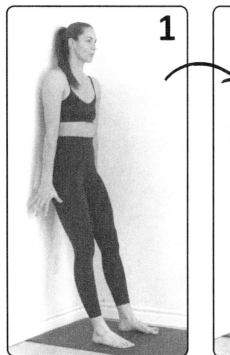

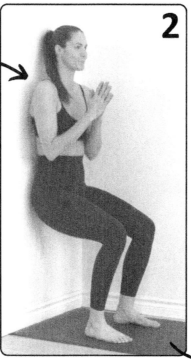

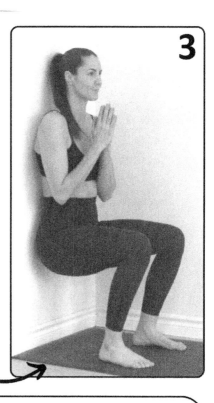

Stand with your back against a wall and your feet hip-width apart, slightly away from the wall.

Lower yourself down until your knees are bent at a 90-degree angle and your thighs are parallel to the ground. Push through your heels to come back up (1) and repeat.

Wall Clamshells

28-Day Challenge
28 | Days 2-9-16-23

BENEFITS

- Strengthens the gluteus medius and minimus, crucial for hip stability.
- Aids in preventing knee and hip injuries by improving lateral hip stability.
- Enhances mobility in the hip joint.

TIPS

- Lie on your side with your hips and shoulders aligned and knees bent at a 90-degree angle. Keep your feet together and pressed against the wall.
- Open your top knee as wide as possible without rotating your hip or pelvis. Return your knee to the starting position with control, maintaining tension in the glutes.
- Common Mistakes: Allowing the hips to roll backward or forward can diminish the effectiveness of the exercise and lead to improper muscle activation.

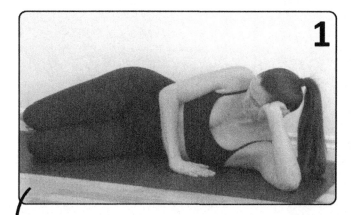

1

Lie on the ground on your left side with your head resting in your hand. Bend your knees at a 90-degree angle. Stack your feet on top of each other with the soles flat against the wall.

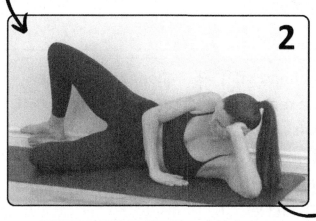

2

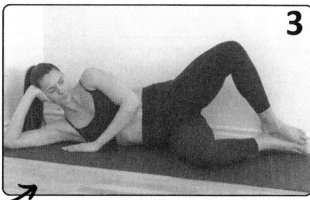

3

Lift your right knee up as high as you can while keeping both feet stacked. Slowly lower your knee back down in a controlled manner. Repeat the exercise, switching the positions of your legs (3).

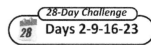
BENEFITS

- Enhances spinal rotation and flexibility.
- Strengthens core and improves shoulder mobility.

TIPS

- Keep core engaged for stability.Focus on the range of motion rather than speed.
- Use your supporting hand to push back to the starting position.
- Ensure even breathing throughout the exercise.
- Common Mistakes: Rushing the movements and not maintaining a straight back can reduce effectiveness.

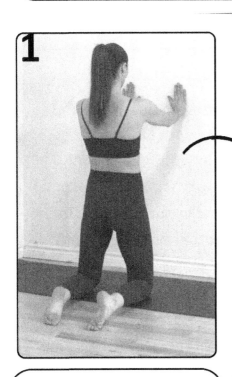

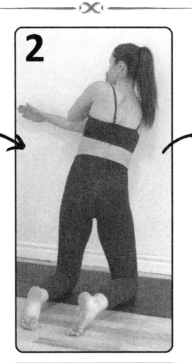

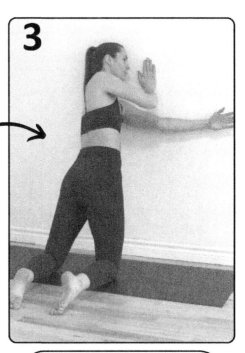

Kneel facing the wall with your knees hip-width apart and your toes flat on the ground. Place your hands on the wall at shoulder level. Maintain this kneeling position with your core engaged and your back straight.

Lift your right hand off the wall and reach under your left arm as far as you can. Push through your left hand to come back up (1).

Repeat, this time reaching with your left hand under your right arm.

Wall Cobra Push Up

BENEFITS

- Strengthens the back, shoulders, and triceps.
- Enhances spinal flexibility and chest opening.
- Promotes core stability.

TIPS

- Ensure your hands are positioned correctly next to your chest for optimal support. Engage your back muscles as you rise to maximize the stretch in your chest and abdominal muscles.
- Maintain a gentle bend in your elbows at the top to avoid locking them.
- Use your breath to guide your movement, inhaling as you rise and exhaling as you lower.

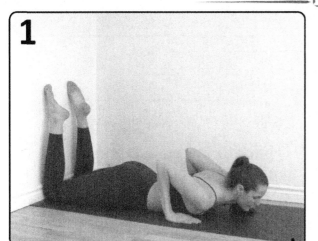

Start on your stomach with knees bent at a 90-degree angle and your shins pressed against the wall. Place your hands flat on the ground next to your chest.

Push through the palms of your hands to come up in a cobra push-up.

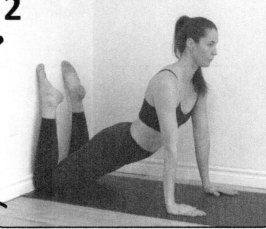

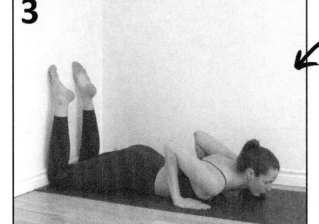

Slowly lower yourself back down in a controlled manner and repeat.

Wall Frog Stretch

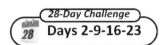

BENEFITS

- Opens and stretches the inner thighs and groin area.
- Enhances hip flexibility and mobility.
- Relieves tension in the lower back through gentle movement.

TIPS

- Begin with your knees wide and feet flexed against the wall to support the stretch.
- Keep your hands positioned under your shoulders to maintain a stable upper body.
- Focus on keeping your lower back straight to avoid strain.
- Common Mistakes: Overextending the knees or pushing too far into discomfort can lead to strain. Ensure the movement is gentle and within a comfortable range.

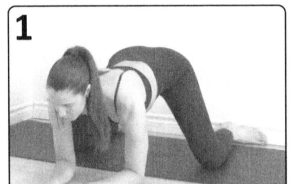

1

Start on the ground with your back to the wall, resting on your hands. Open your knees as wide as possible and place your feet on the wall.

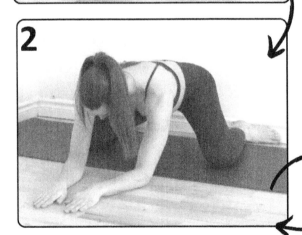

2

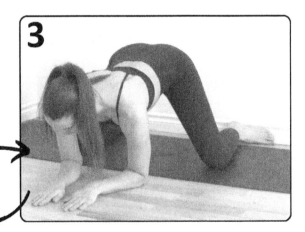

3

Rock your body backward and forward while keeping your lower back straight. Feel the stretch in your hips.

Days 3-10-17-24: Elevating Your Wall Pilates Practice

Welcome to Day 3 of your 28-day Wall Pilates challenge, where we continue to build strength, flexibility, and balance through a series of targeted exercises. Today, you'll engage in a dynamic routine designed to further challenge your body while ensuring you maintain the joy of movement. Let's explore the workouts for today:

Warm-Up: Wall Quad Stretch

Begin your session with the _Wall Quad Stretch_ to loosen up your quadriceps and hip flexors, ensuring these key muscles are prepped for the day's activities. This stretch is essential for maintaining lower body flexibility and preventing tightness.

Core: Wall Assisted Plank & Wall Mountain Climbers

Strengthen your core foundation with the _Wall Assisted Plank_, an exercise that promotes core stability and endurance.

Ramp up the intensity with _Wall Mountain Climbers_, which not only engages your entire core but also introduces a cardiovascular element to your workout, boosting your heart rate and improving overall fitness.

Lower Body: Standing Hip Abduction, Wall Plié Squat with Heel Lifts, Wall Plié Squat Pulses, Wall Sit with Heel Lifts

Activate your outer thighs and glutes with _Standing Hip Abduction_, enhancing hip mobility and lateral strength.

Incorporate _Wall Plié Squat with Heel Lifts_ and _Wall Plié Squat Pulses_ for a deep engagement of your glutes, thighs, and calves, further emphasized by the added challenge of heel lifts for calf strengthening.

Finish your lower body segment with _Wall Sit with Heel Lifts_, combining endurance and strength for a comprehensive lower body workout.

Upper Body: Wall Kneeling Child's Pose & Wall Kneeling Push Up

Transition to upper body work with a combination of stretching and strengthening. Start with the _Wall Kneeling Child's Pose_ to stretch your shoulders, chest, and back.

Follow up with _Wall Kneeling Push Ups_ to build strength in your chest, shoulders, and arms, promoting upper body muscle tone and endurance.

Cool-Down: Standing Forward Fold

Conclude today's routine with the _Standing Forward Fold_, a soothing stretch that relaxes your spine, shoulders, and hamstrings. This pose helps to calm your mind and body, rounding off your workout on a peaceful note. As you move through Day 3, each workout should be performed for **1 minute**, culminating in a **10-minute routine** that balances strength, flexibility, and mental focus.

Wall Quad Stretch - Left

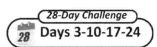

28-Day Challenge
28 Days 3-10-17-24

BENEFITS

- Stretches and loosens the quadriceps muscles.
- Aids in reducing tightness in the front thigh area.
- Can help prevent quad-related strains and improve flexibility.

TIPS

- Use the wall for balance and support during the stretch.
- Pull your leg gently to avoid overstretching or causing discomfort.
- Keep your standing leg slightly bent to maintain stability.
- Engage your core and maintain an upright posture.
- Common Mistakes: Overarching the lower back or tilting the hips can decrease the effectiveness of the stretch and risk injury.

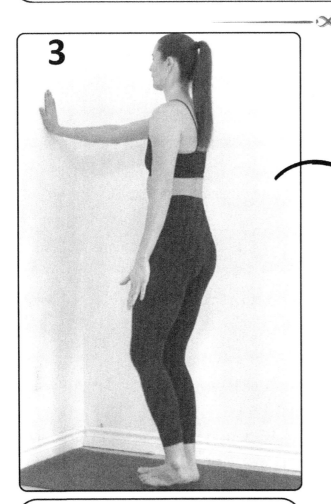

**Stand with your feet hip-width apart facing the wall.
Place your right hand on the wall.**

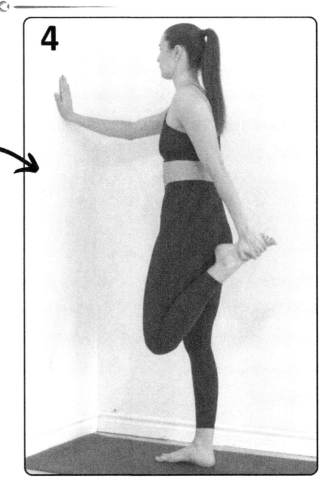

**Bend your left leg and hold your left toes with your left hand.
Gently pull your left leg up while using the wall for support.**

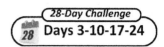
BENEFITS

- Stretches and loosens the quadriceps muscles.
- Aids in reducing tightness in the front thigh area.
- Can help prevent quad-related strains and improve flexibility.

TIPS

- Use the wall for balance and support during the stretch.
- Pull your leg gently to avoid overstretching or causing discomfort.
- Keep your standing leg slightly bent to maintain stability.
- Engage your core and maintain an upright posture.
- Common Mistakes: Overarching the lower back or tilting the hips can decrease the effectiveness of the stretch and risk injury.

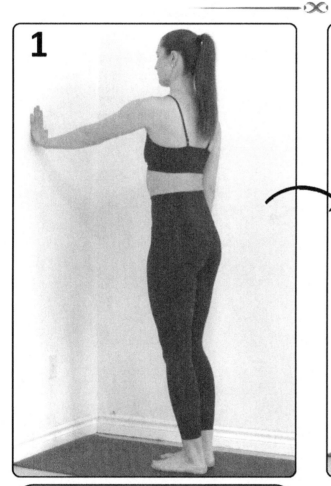

1

Stand with your feet hip-width apart facing the wall. Place your left hand on the wall.

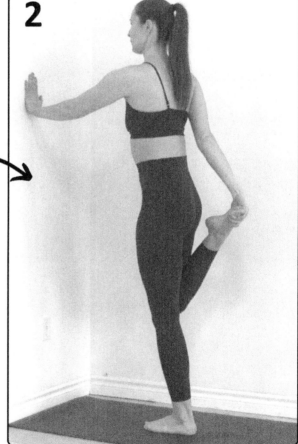

2

Bend your right leg and hold your right toes with your right hand. Gently pull your right leg up while using the wall for support.

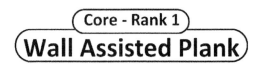

Core - Rank 1
Wall Assisted Plank

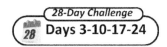
28-Day Challenge
28 Days 3-10-17-24

BENEFITS

- Strengthens the core, including the abdominals and lower back.
- Improves posture and stability.
- Serves as an introduction to more challenging plank variations.

TIPS

- Engage your core to prevent sagging or arching in the lower back.
- Keep the neck in a neutral position.
- Focus on breathing steadily to maintain the pose.
- Common Mistakes: Allowing the hips to rise or drop can compromise the effectiveness and increase the risk of strain.

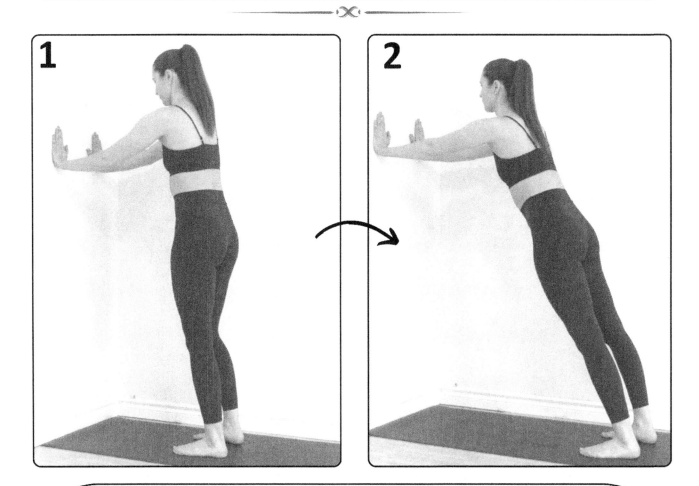

Stand facing the wall with your feet hip-width apart. Place your hands on the wall at chest level. Step your feet back one step. Hold this position by keeping your core engaged and back straight.

Wall Mountain Climbers

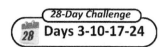

BENEFITS

- Enhances core strength and stability.
- Increases cardiovascular endurance.
- Improves coordination and agility.

TIPS

- Maintain a strong plank position with the core engaged throughout the exercise. Drive knees towards the chest with control, focusing on engaging the lower abs.
- Keep the movement rhythmic, alternating legs smoothly.
- Ensure hands remain firmly placed on the wall to support your body weight.
- Common Mistakes: Allowing the hips to sag or lift can reduce core engagement and the overall effectiveness of the exercise.

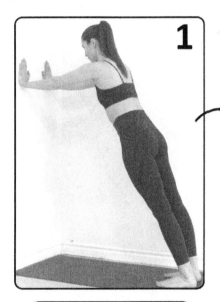

1

Stand facing the wall with your feet hip-width apart. Place your hands on the wall at chest level. Step your feet back one step. Hold this position by keeping your core engaged and back straight.

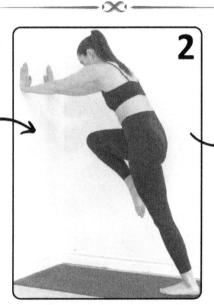

2

From here, lift your right foot up and drive your knee towards your chest.

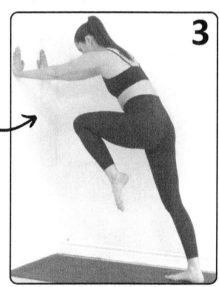

3

Lower your right foot back down and repeat on the left side

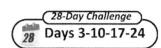

BENEFITS

- Strengthens the muscles of the outer thigh and glutes.
- Improves hip stability and balance.
- Enhances lateral movement coordination.

TIPS

- Use the wall for balance, keeping the supporting arm lightly pressed for stability. Engage your core throughout the exercise to maintain upright posture.
- Lift your leg to the side with control, focusing on the abduction movement. Keep the movement of the lifted leg smooth and controlled, avoiding any jerky motions.
- Common Mistakes: Leaning too far into the wall or compensating by tilting the upper body can reduce the effectiveness of the hip abduction. Ensure the lifting leg moves independently, without swinging.

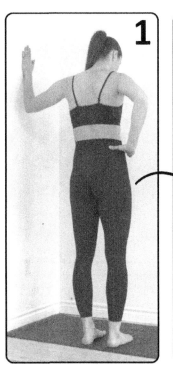
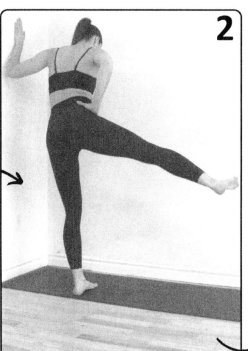
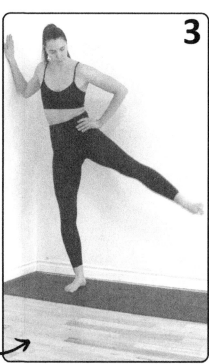

Stand next to the wall. Place your left hand on the wall and put your right hand on your hip.

Keep your core engaged and shift your weight onto your left leg. Lift your right leg out to the side, then slowly lower it back down in a controlled manner (1).Do the same on the other side (3), placing the right hand on the wall and the left hand on the hip. Lift the left leg out to the side then slowly lower it back down.

Wall Plié Squat with Heel Lifts

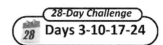

28-Day Challenge
28 Days 3-10-17-24

BENEFITS

- Strengthens the calves, quadriceps, glutes, and inner thighs.
- Enhances lower body stability and balance.
- Improves ankle mobility and flexibility.

TIPS

- Maintain a deep plié squat position, ensuring knees are aligned with toes.
- Lift your heels as high as possible while keeping the squat depth constant.
- Lower the heels with control to engage the calf muscles fully.
- Common Mistakes: Losing the squat depth while lifting the heels or allowing knees to collapse inward can reduce the effectiveness of the exercise and risk injury.

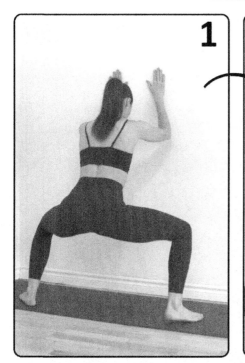

1

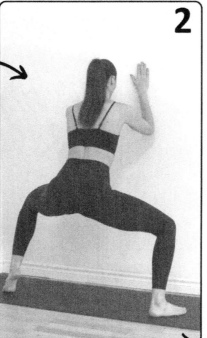

2

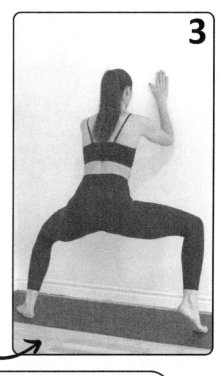

3

Stand facing the wall with your feet in a wide stance and your feet externally rotated. Place your hands on the wall.

Squat down until your knees are at a 90-degree angle and hold this position. Raise both heels up and down for the duration of this exercise.

Wall Plié Squat Pulses

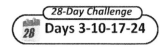
BENEFITS

- Targets the inner thighs, glutes, and quadriceps.
- Enhances lower body strength and endurance.
- Improves flexibility and balance.

TIPS

- Keep your feet turned out and wide apart to maximize inner thigh engagement. Pulse gently in the squat position, focusing on engaging your muscles with each movement.
- Ensure your knees track over your toes and avoid extending past your feet.
- Common Mistakes: Rising too high out of the squat position between pulses can lessen the exercise's intensity, and losing the depth of the squat can reduce its effectiveness.

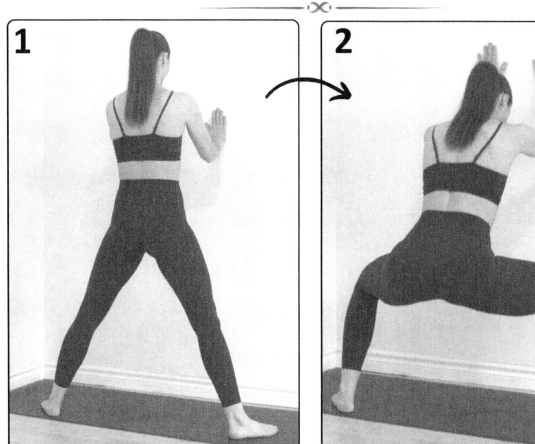

Stand facing the wall with your feet in a wide stance and your feet externally rotated. Place your hands on the wall. Squat down until your knees are at a 90-degree angle and your thighs are parallel with the ground. Hold this position and perform small pulses. Push through your heels to come back up (1).

Wall Sit with Heel Lifts

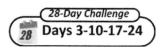

28-Day Challenge
Days 3-10-17-24

BENEFITS

- Strengthens the quadriceps, calves, and glutes.
- Enhances lower body endurance and stability.
- Improves balance and ankle mobility.

TIPS

- Ensure your back is flat against the wall throughout the exercise for support. Keep your knees bent at a 90-degree angle, directly above your ankles.
- Lift your heels smoothly, focusing on the calf muscles, and then lower them with control. Maintain the wall sit posture without changing the angle of your knees as you perform the heel lifts.
- Breathe evenly throughout the exercise to maintain posture and stability.
- Common Mistakes: Shifting too much weight onto the toes can lead to balance issues.

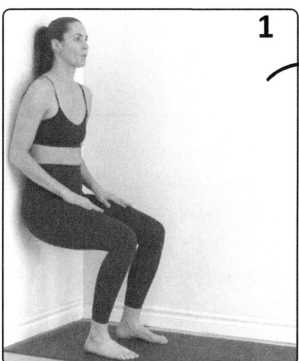

1

Stand with your back against a wall and your feet hip-width apart, slightly away from the wall. Squat down until your knees are bent at a 90-degree angle.

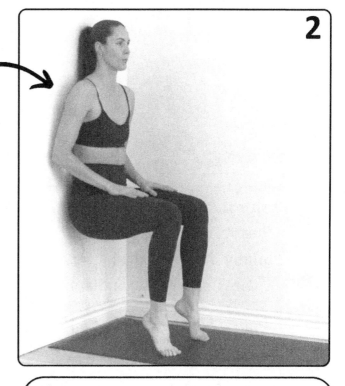

2

While sitting in this position, lift your heels up as high as you can go, hold briefly, then slowly lower them back down and repeat.

Wall Kneeling Child's Pose

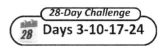

BENEFITS

- Stretches the chest, shoulders, and arms.
- Encourages relaxation and release of upper body tension.
- Promotes a gentle stretch in the lower back and hips.

TIPS

- Keep your hands at shoulder level to ensure an effective stretch. Focus on pushing the hips back to deepen the stretch in the shoulders and chest.
- Hold the position briefly to allow your muscles to relax and stretch.
- Move in and out of the stretch with controlled, gentle motions.
- Common Mistakes: Not maintaining a stable hand position can lessen the stretch's effectiveness, and rushing the movement may prevent the full benefits of the stretch.

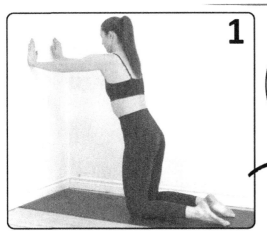

1

Start in a kneeling position facing the wall. Place your hands on the wall at shoulder level. Step yourself back one step.

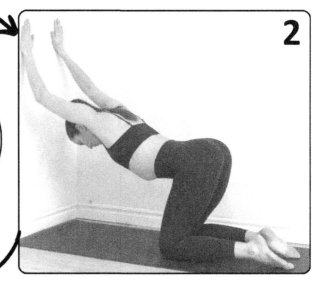

2

Push your hips back and bring your chest towards the ground. Hold briefly, feeling a stretch in your chest, shoulders, and arms.

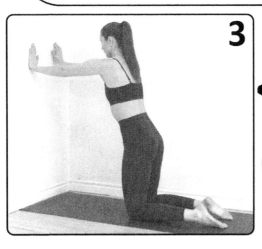

3

Return to the starting position and repeat.

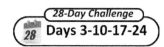
Wall Kneeling Push Up

BENEFITS

- Strengthens the chest, shoulders, and triceps.
- Engages the core, promoting good posture.
- Serves as an introduction to more advanced push-up variations.

TIPS

- Keep a neutral spine and engaged core throughout the exercise.
- Ensure elbows bend at a 45-degree angle to the body to protect the joints.
- Common Mistakes: Not aligning hands at shoulder level can place undue stress on the shoulders, and flaring elbows out too wide can compromise form.

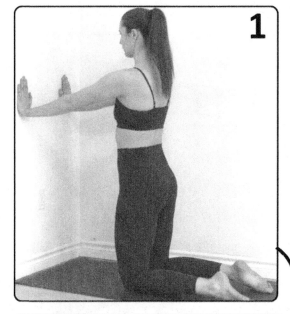

1

Kneel facing the wall with your knees hip-width apart and your toes flat on the ground. Place your hands on the wall at shoulder level.Maintain this kneeling position with your core engaged and your back straight.

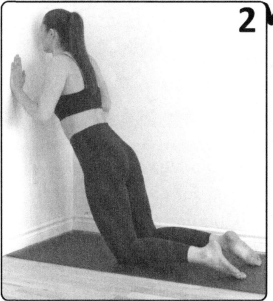

2

Bend your elbows and lower your upper body towards the wall, bringing your chest closer to it. Push through the palms of your hands to return to the starting position and repeat.

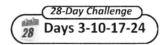
BENEFITS

- Stretches the hamstrings and lower back, promoting flexibility.
- Can relieve tension in the upper body when performed gently.
- Enhances circulation by inverting the torso.

TIPS

- Keep a slight bend in your knees to avoid strain on the lower back and hamstrings.
- Let your head hang freely to release neck tension.
- Breathe deeply in the position, allowing each exhale to help you deepen the stretch.
- Common Mistakes: Locking the knees or rounding the back too much can lead to discomfort and reduce the effectiveness of the stretch.

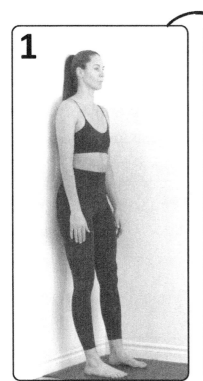

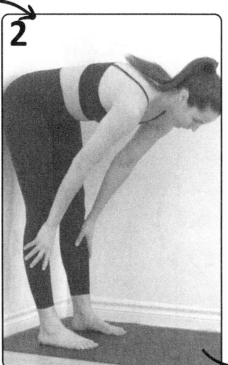

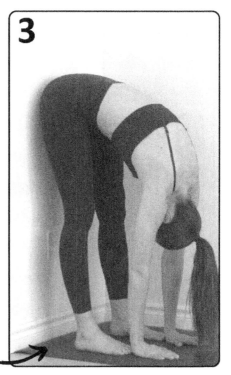

Start in a standing position with your back against the wall and your feet slightly away from the wall.

Bend at the torso to bring your upper body down and reach for your feet with your hands. Hold this position to feel a stretch in your hamstrings.

Days 4-11-18-25: Strengthening and Stretching with Wall Pilates

Welcome to Day 4 of your transformative 28-day Wall Pilates challenge. Today's routine is carefully designed to enhance your strength, balance, and flexibility.

Warm-Up: Thoracic Rotations

Kick off your session with *Thoracic Rotations*, a pivotal movement to increase spinal mobility and reduce tension in your upper back. This exercise is fundamental for a healthy posture and ease of movement in daily activities.

Core: Wall Cross Body Mountain Climbers & Wall Elevated Plank

Intensify your core workout with *Wall Cross Body Mountain Climbers*, targeting your obliques and bringing a cardio element to your routine for enhanced fat burn and agility. Stabilize and strengthen your core with the *Wall Elevated Plank*. This variation challenges your abdominal muscles, promoting endurance and a solid core foundation vital for overall fitness and well-being.

Lower Body: Wall Glute Bridges | Clamshells, Wall Single Leg Glute Bridge, Wall Side Lunges

Elevate your lower body workout with a series of glute-focused exercises. *Wall Glute Bridges* and their variations, *including Clamshells* and *Single Leg Glute Bridge*, concentrate on your glutes and hamstrings, crucial for lower body strength, stability, and injury prevention. Incorporate *Wall Side Lunges* to work your inner and outer thighs, enhancing your leg strength and flexibility, an essential aspect of a balanced fitness regimen.

Upper Body: Wall Single Arm Triceps Press & Wall Diamond Push Up

Target your upper body with the *Wall Single Arm Triceps Press*, focusing on your triceps for toned arms and improved upper body strength. The *Wall Diamond Push Up* further sculpts your chest, shoulders, and triceps, promoting muscle definition and strength essential for a powerful upper body.

Cool-Down: Wall Standing Child's Pose

End your session feeling relaxed and rejuvenated with the *Wall Standing Child's Pose*, a gentle stretch that releases tension in your back, shoulders, and neck.

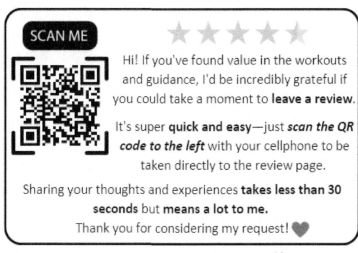

SCAN ME

★ ★ ★ ★ ★

Hi! If you've found value in the workouts and guidance, I'd be incredibly grateful if you could take a moment to **leave a review.**

It's super **quick and easy**—just *scan the QR code to the left* with your cellphone to be taken directly to the review page.

Sharing your thoughts and experiences **takes less than 30 seconds** but **means a lot to me.**
Thank you for considering my request! ♥

Wall Thoracic Rotations

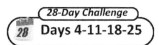

28-Day Challenge
28 Days 4-11-18-25

BENEFITS

- Enhances mid-back (thoracic spine) mobility.
- Encourages rotational flexibility and range of motion.
- Helps release tension in the upper back and shoulders.

TIPS

- Keep your feet planted and hip-width apart for stable rotation.
- Rotate from the mid-back, keeping the hips square to avoid over-rotation. Use gentle pressure against the wall to deepen the stretch without forcing it.
- Alternate sides smoothly to work on balanced flexibility.
- Common Mistakes: Rotating primarily from the hips or shoulders rather than the thoracic spine can reduce the effectiveness of the exercise.

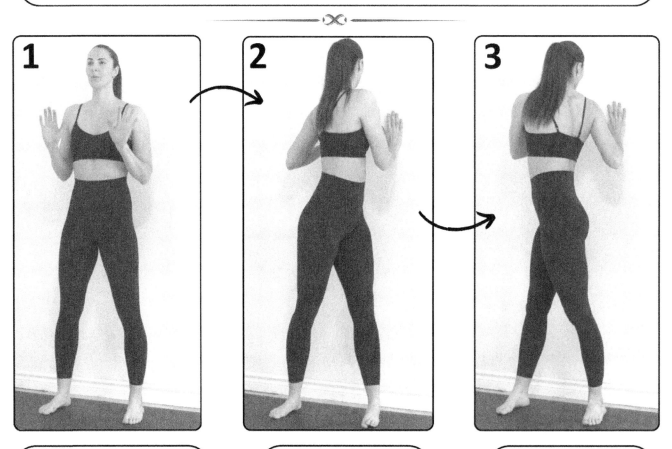

1 Stand facing away from the wall with your feet hip-width apart. Bring your hands up to chest level.

2 Rotate your torso to the left and place your hands on the wall.

3 Gently push your body away (1) and rotate your torso to the other side (3). Alternate between sides

Wall Cross Body Mountain Climbers

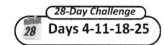

BENEFITS

- Targets and strengthens the core, with a focus on the obliques.
- Improves cardiovascular endurance and promotes fat burning.
- Enhances coordination and agility through cross-body movement.

TIPS

- Maintain a strong, engaged core to stabilize your body and enhance the twist. Aim for controlled knee drives, focusing on bringing the knee across the body. Keep a steady pace to maintain form and maximize cardiovascular benefits.
- Ensure hands are firmly pressed against the wall to support your weight.
- Common Mistakes: Losing the plank form by sagging the hips or piking up can diminish the exercise's effectiveness and risk strain.

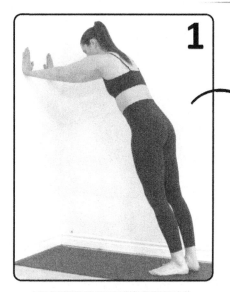

1

Stand facing the wall with your feet hip-width apart. Place your hands on the wall at chest level. Step your feet back one step. Hold this position by keeping your core engaged and back straight.

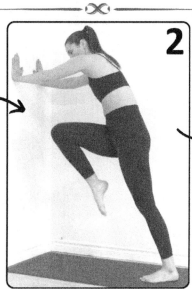

2

From here, drive your right knee towards the left side of your body.

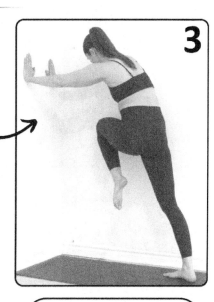

3

Lower your right leg back down and repeat, this time driving your left knee towards the right side of your body.

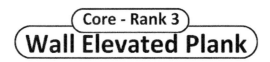

Core - Rank 3
Wall Elevated Plank

28-Day Challenge
Days 4-11-18-25

BENEFITS

- Significantly strengthens the core, including the abdominals and lower back.
- Engages the shoulders, glutes, and quads for full-body activation.
- Improves posture and stability through enhanced core control.

TIPS

- Ensure wrists are directly under shoulders for optimal support and alignment. Press feet firmly against the wall to stabilize and intensify the plank.
- Keep a straight line from head to heels, focusing on a tight core and engaged glutes. Breathe steadily to maintain posture and endurance throughout the hold.
- Common Mistakes: Allowing the hips to sag or pike can compromise form and reduce effectiveness. Ensure consistent engagement across all muscle groups.

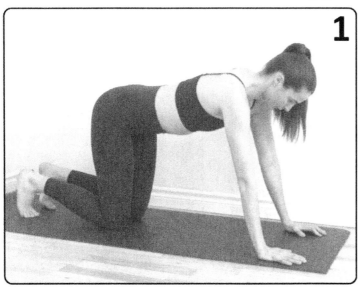

1

Start on all fours facing away from the wall.

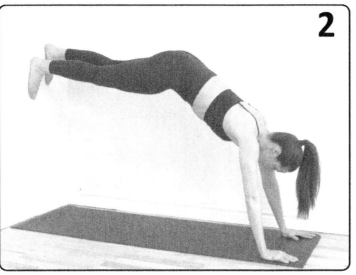

2

Place your feet on the wall, with your wrists under your shoulders. Hold this position while keeping your shoulder blades, core, glutes, and quads engaged.

56

Wall Glute Bridges

BENEFITS

- Strengthens the glutes, hamstrings, and lower back.
- Enhances hip mobility and stability.
- Can alleviate lower back pain by improving core and posterior chain strength.

TIPS

- Ensure your feet are planted firmly against the wall and spaced hip-width apart. Drive through your heels to lift your hips, focusing on engaging your glutes fully at the top.
- Keep the movement slow and controlled, maximizing muscle activation.
- Aim to create a straight line from your knees to your shoulders at the top of the movement.
- Common Mistakes: Arching the lower back excessively or not engaging the core can reduce the effectiveness and potentially strain the back.

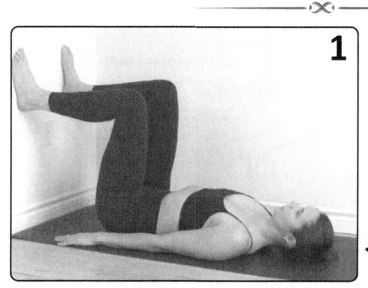

1

Lie on the ground with your feet on the wall. Keep your knees bent at a 90-degree angle.

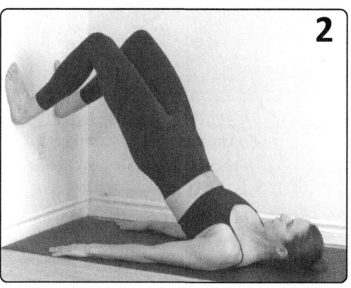

2

Push through your heels to lift your hips up, squeezing your glutes at the top of this movement. Slowly lower your hips back down (1).

Wall Glute Bridges with Clamshells

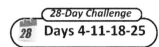
28-Day Challenge
Days 4-11-18-25

BENEFITS

- Targets and strengthens the glutes, inner thighs, and pelvic floor.
- Improves hip mobility and stability.
- Enhances core engagement and lower back support.

TIPS

- Press firmly through your heels on the wall to activate your glutes and hamstrings effectively. Focus on lifting your hips as high as comfortably possible to deepen the engagement of the glute muscles.
- As you open your knees, maintain control and engage your inner thighs to maximize the benefit of the clamshell movement.
- Ensure a smooth transition between lifting, opening the knees, and lowering back down to foster continuous muscle engagement and avoid any jerky movements.

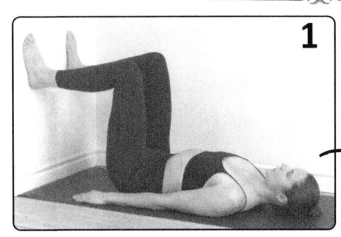

1

Lie on the ground with your feet on the wall. Keep your knees bent at a 90-degree angle.

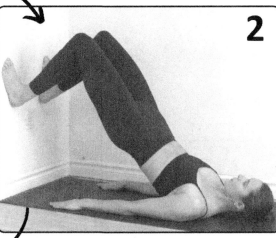

2

Push through your heels to lift your hips up.

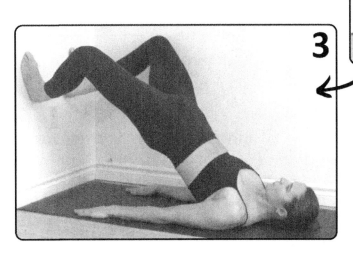

3

Once you've reached your highest position, open your knees out to the side. Bring them back in and slowly lower your hips back down (1).

Wall Single Leg Glute Bridge

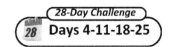

BENEFITS

- Isolates and strengthens the glutes and hamstrings on each side, promoting muscular balance.
- Enhances hip stability and unilateral strength.
- Improves core stability and lower back support.

TIPS

- Keep the foot on the wall firmly planted and focus on pushing through the heel for maximum glute activation.
- Extend the opposite leg towards the ceiling to maintain alignment and challenge stability. Squeeze the glute of the working leg at the top of the movement for an extra contraction.
- Ensure a controlled ascent and descent to maintain engagement and protect the lower back.
- Common Mistakes: Dropping the hips unevenly or losing control can reduce the exercise's effectiveness and risk strain. Ensure the non-working leg remains straight and engaged.

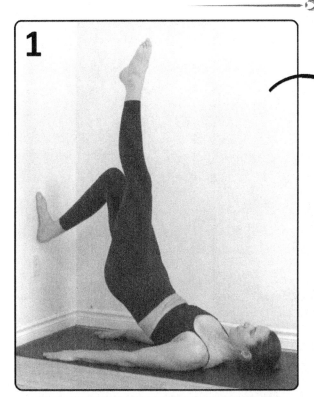

1

Lie on the ground with your feet on the wall. Extend your left leg, pointing it towards the sky. Push through your right heel to lift your hips up, squeezing your glute at the top of this movement.

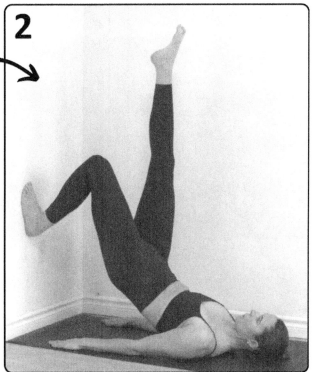

2

Lie on the ground with your feet on the wall. Extend your right leg, pointing it towards the sky. Push through your left heel to lift your hips up, squeezing your glute at the top of this movement.

Wall Side Lunges

BENEFITS

- Strengthens the muscles in the thighs, particularly the adductors and glutes.
- Enhances hip flexibility and mobility.
- Improves balance and lower body stability.

TIPS

- Aim to keep the bent knee in line with your foot, avoiding it extending past your toes.
- Maintain the straight leg with the foot firmly planted.
- Push through the heel of the bent leg to return to the starting position, engaging your glutes. Alternate sides to ensure balanced strength and flexibility in both legs.
- Common Mistakes: Allowing the knee of the bent leg to collapse inward can strain the knee joint, and not keeping the hips back can reduce the effectiveness of the stretch on the inner thigh.

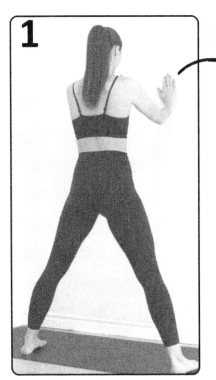 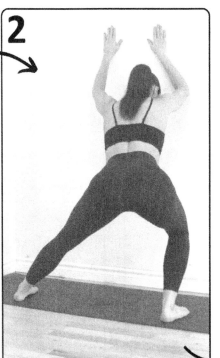 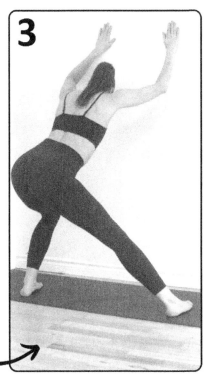

Stand facing the wall with your feet in a wide stance. Place your hands on the wall for support.

Hinge your hips back and bend your right knee to a 90-degree angle while keeping your left leg straight. Push through your right heel to come back up. Repeat the exercise with the left leg.

Wall Single Arm Triceps Press - Left

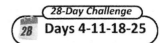

28-Day Challenge
2B Days 4-11-18-25

BENEFITS

- Isolates and strengthens the left tricep muscle.
- Enhances unilateral upper body strength and balance.
- Engages core muscles to maintain stability.

TIPS

- Stand arm's length from the wall for optimal positioning.
- Keep your feet firmly planted and your body straight as you lower and raise yourself.
- Focus on using your tricep to press back up, avoiding momentum.
- Keep movements controlled and steady to target the tricep effectively.
- Common Mistakes: Moving too quickly or not keeping the elbow close to the body can reduce isolation of the tricep muscle.

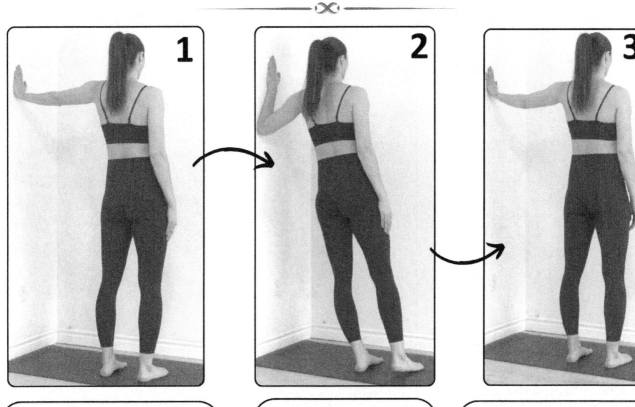

1 Stand next to the wall, an arm's length away. Place your left hand on the wall while keeping your arm straight.

2 From there, lower yourself until your elbow touches the wall.

3 Push through the palm of your hand to push yourself back up, activating your triceps as you come up.

Wall Single Arm Triceps Press - Right

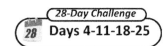

BENEFITS

- Isolates and strengthens the right tricep muscle.
- Enhances unilateral upper body strength and balance.
- Engages core muscles to maintain stability.

TIPS

- Stand arm's length from the wall for optimal positioning.
- Keep your feet firmly planted and your body straight as you lower and raise yourself.
- Focus on using your tricep to press back up, avoiding momentum.
- Keep movements controlled and steady to target the tricep effectively.
- Common Mistakes: Moving too quickly or not keeping the elbow close to the body can reduce isolation of the tricep muscle.

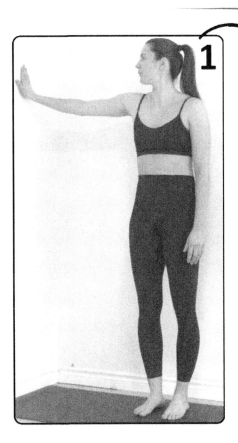

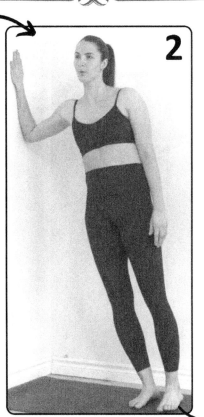

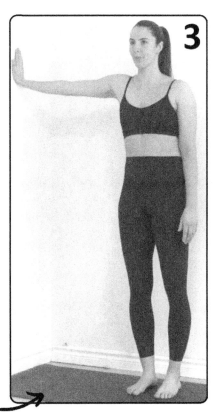

Stand next to the wall, an arm's length away. Place your right hand on the wall while keeping your arm straight.

From there, lower yourself until your elbow touches the wall.

Push through the palm of your hand to push yourself back up, activating your triceps as you come up.

Wall Diamond Push Ups

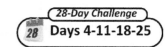

BENEFITS

- Targets the triceps and the inner chest muscles.
- Promotes muscle definition.
- Engages the core for improved stability and posture.

TIPS

- Form a diamond shape with your fingers to properly target the triceps and inner chest.
- Keep the core engaged and maintain a straight line from head to heels.
- Lower with control and push back up with emphasis on the triceps.
- Ensure elbows point back and down, not out to the sides.
- Common Mistakes: Placing hands too high or too low on the wall can compromise form and effectiveness.

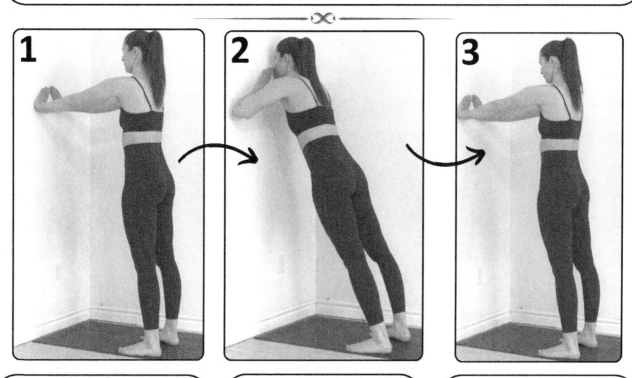

1 Stand facing the wall with your feet hip-width apart. Place your hands on the wall at shoulder level, creating a diamond shape with your fingers. Step your feet back one step. Hold this position by keeping your core engaged.

2 Bend your elbows and lower yourself to bring your chest towards the wall.

3 Push through the palms of your hands to come back up and repeat.

Wall Standing Child's Pose

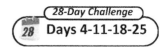

28-Day Challenge
28 Days 4-11-18-25

BENEFITS

- Stretches the shoulders, chest, and upper back.
- Encourages relaxation and release of tension.
- Mimics the traditional Child's Pose, providing a gentle inversion.

TIPS

- Push your hips back as you lower your chest to deepen the stretch.
- Keep your arms straight and your head in line with your arms.
- Hold the stretch to allow your muscles to relax and open up.
- Common Mistakes: Avoid lifting the heels or arching the lower back, which can reduce the effectiveness of the stretch.

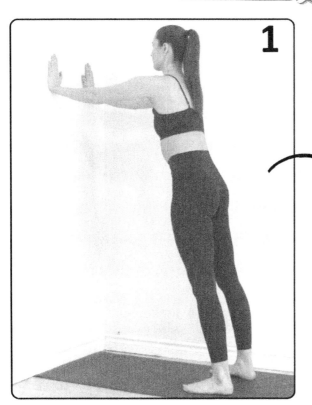

1

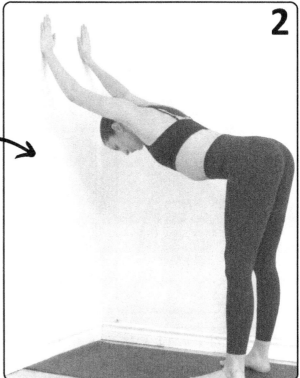

2

Stand facing the wall with your feet shoulder-width apart. Place your hands on the wall at shoulder level. Step your feet back one step.

While keeping your hands in the same position, push your hips back and bring your chest towards the ground. Hold briefly, feeling a stretch in your chest, shoulders, and arms, then return to the starting position and repeat.

Days 5-12-19-26: Full-Body Engagement with Precision

Welcome to Day 5 of the 28-Day Wall Pilates challenge. Each exercise today is designed to engage your entire body with a focus on precision and mindfulness, ensuring you benefit maximally from every movement. Let's explore today's routine:

Warm-Up: Wall Chest Stretch

Begin your day with a *Wall Chest Stretch*, essential for opening up the chest and shoulders. This stretch not only prepares your upper body for the exercises ahead but also helps alleviate any tension from daily activities, promoting better posture and breathing.

Core: Plank Wall Taps & Wall Cross Body Toe Touches Crunches

Activate your core with *Plank Wall Taps*, a dynamic exercise that challenges your stability and strengthens your abdominal muscles. It's an excellent way to kickstart your metabolism and engage the core from different angles.

Transition to *Wall Cross Body Toe Touches Crunches* for a focused core workout that targets your obliques and abs. This exercise enhances coordination and balance, vital for core stability and functional movement.

Lower Body: Wall Marching Glute Bridge, Wall Walking Glute Bridge, Wall Glute Kickbacks, Wall Elevated Split Squat

Strengthen your lower body with a series of glute and leg exercises. The *Wall Marching Glute Bridge* and *Wall Walking Glute Bridge* are perfect for activating your glutes and hamstrings, essential for lower body power and stability. Add intensity with *Wall Glute Kickbacks*, focusing on glute engagement for a toned and strong backside. Incorporate *Wall Elevated Split Squat* to target your quads and improve lower body strength and flexibility.

Upper Body: Wall Arm Angels & Wall Arm Butterflies

For the upper body, *Wall Arm Angels* and *Wall Arm Butterflies* offer a gentle yet effective way to stretch and strengthen the shoulders, upper back, and arms. These exercises improve mobility and reduce the risk of shoulder injuries, enhancing your overall upper body health.

Cool-Down: Wall Reclined Pigeon

Finish your session with *Wall Reclined Pigeon*, a deep stretch that targets the hips and lower back. This cool-down exercise alleviates tension and promotes flexibility, ensuring you conclude your workout feeling relaxed and revitalized.

Day 5's routine, with a total of **10 minutes** of targeted exercises, is a testament to the holistic approach of Wall Pilates. Each workout is performed for **1 minute**, emphasizing form and function to bring about significant benefits to your body. From enhancing core strength to improving flexibility and reducing stiffness, today's exercises are pivotal in your fitness journey. Keep focused, maintain consistency, and watch as you transform with each day's practice.

Wall Chest Stretch

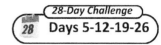
BENEFITS

- Opens and stretches the chest and shoulder muscles.
- Improves posture and mobility in the upper body.
- Relieves tightness from sitting or repetitive upper body activities.

TIPS

- Maintain a 90-degree angle in your elbow to target the chest and shoulder stretch effectively.
- Gently rotate away from the wall to increase the stretch without straining.
- Keep your feet firmly planted and your body upright.
- Hold the stretch for several deep breaths, allowing the muscles to release tension.
- Common Mistakes: Over-rotating the body or not keeping the forearm in contact with the wall can diminish the stretch's benefits.

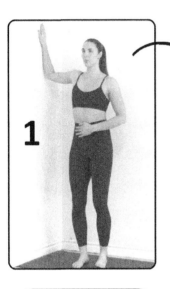

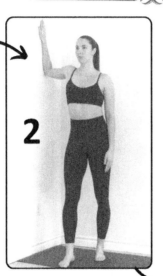

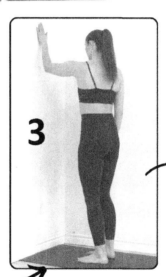

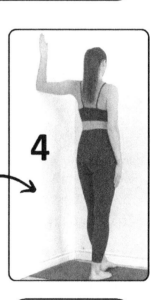

1 — Stand facing a wall with your feet shoulder-width apart. Bend your right arm at a 90-degree angle and place your forearm on the wall.

2 — Turn your body to the left, maintaining contact with the wall. Feel the stretch in your chest and right shoulder

3 — Stand facing a wall with your feet shoulder-width apart. Bend your left arm at a 90-degree angle and place your forearm on the wall.

4 — Turn your body to the right, maintaining contact with the wall. Feel the stretch in your chest and left shoulder.

Plank Wall Taps

BENEFITS

- Enhances core stability by challenging balance and control.
- Strengthens the shoulders and arms through dynamic movement.
- Improves coordination and engages the entire body.

TIPS

- Maintain a strong plank position with hips squared to the ground.
- Shift your weight carefully to maintain balance as you tap the wall.
- Keep your core engaged to prevent the hips from sagging or rotating.
- Focus on smooth, controlled taps to maximize muscle engagement.
- Common Mistakes: Losing plank form by letting the back arch or hips rise can reduce the effectiveness and risk strain.

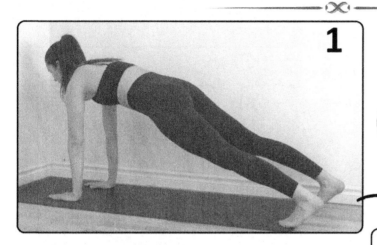

1

Start in a high plank position facing the wall. Keep your hips squared to the ground.

2

Shift your weight onto your right hand while tapping the wall with your left hand. Bring your left hand back down (1).

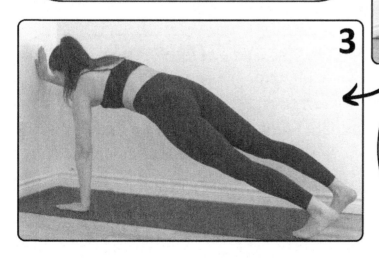

3

Shift your weight to your left hand and tap the wall with your right hand. Continue alternating sides while keeping your core engaged and your back straight.

Wall Cross Body Toe Touches Crunches

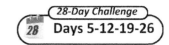

28-Day Challenge
28 Days 5-12-19-26

BENEFITS

- Targets and strengthens the obliques and abdominal muscles.
- Enhances flexibility and range of motion in the legs.
- Improves coordination between upper and lower body movements.

TIPS

- Keep your legs straight and pressed against the wall to maintain proper form.
- Focus on lifting your shoulder off the ground to reach your toes, engaging the core.
- Alternate sides smoothly, ensuring equal work on both sides of the body. Keep the movement controlled, emphasizing the crunch and reach.
- Common Mistakes: Pulling on the neck instead of using core strength to lift, and bending the knees, which can reduce the effectiveness of the exercise.

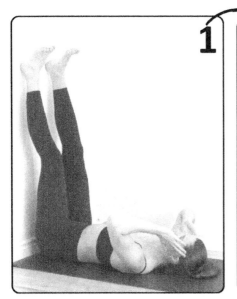

1

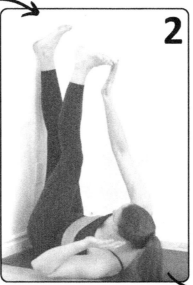

2

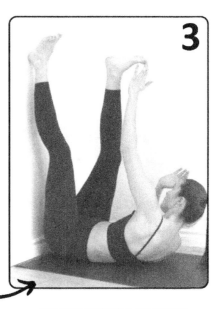

3

Lie on the ground with your legs up the wall. Keep your legs straight. Bend your elbows and place your hands by the sides of your head.

Bring your left leg towards yourself, and reach your left toes with your right hand.

Return to the starting position and repeat, this time bringing your right leg towards yourself and reaching with your left hand.

Wall Marching Glute Bridge

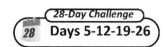

28-Day Challenge
Days 5-12-19-26

BENEFITS

- Strengthens the glutes and hamstrings while engaging the core.
- Improves hip mobility and stability.
- Enhances coordination and balance in a static hold position.

TIPS

- Ensure your hips remain lifted and stable throughout the exercise to maintain tension in the glutes.
- Move each leg with control, focusing on maintaining the height of your hips without rocking. Alternate legs smoothly, ensuring an even pace and distribution of movement.
- Common Mistakes: Dropping the hips during the march or losing the engagement of the glutes can reduce the effectiveness of the exercise.

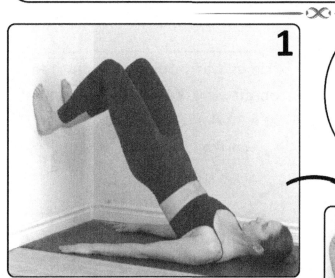

1

Lie on the ground with your feet on the wall. Keep your knees bent at a 90-degree angle. Push through your heels to lift your hips up and hold this position.

2

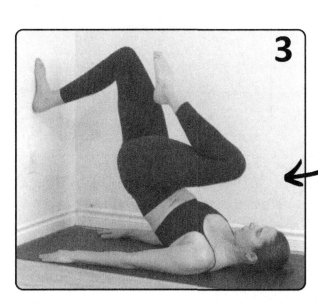

3

Drive one knee towards your chest at a time while keeping everything else stable.

Wall Walking Glute Bridge

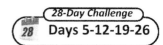

28-Day Challenge
28 Days 5-12-19-26

BENEFITS

- Enhances glute and hamstring strength with dynamic movement.
- Promotes core stability and hip mobility.
- Increases endurance and control in the elevated hip position.

TIPS

- Keep your core engaged and hips elevated throughout the exercise to maximize glute activation.
- Move your feet up and down the wall with controlled, deliberate steps, maintaining steady hip height.
- Focus on smooth transitions to keep the movement fluid and stable.
- Common Mistakes: Allowing the hips to sag during the walk can diminish the exercise's effectiveness and place undue strain on the lower back.

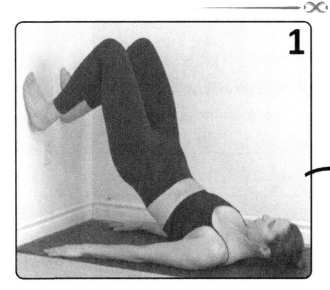

1

Lie on the ground with your feet on the wall. Keep your knees bent at a 90-degree angle. Engage your core and lift your hips up.

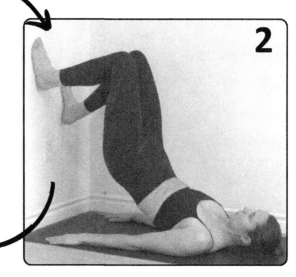

2

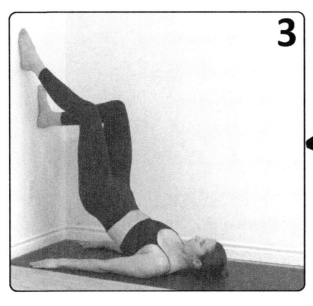

3

While keeping your hips up, slowly start walking your feet up and down the wall.

Wall Glute Kickbacks

BENEFITS

- Targets and strengthens the glutes, enhancing buttock shape and power.
- Improves lower back stability.
- Aids in the correction of muscular imbalances and enhances posture.

TIPS

- Maintain a slight bend in your standing leg for stability.
- Focus on a controlled, powerful kickback, engaging the glutes at the top of the movement. Keep your back flat and avoid arching your lower back as you kick back.
- Common Mistakes: Rushing the movement or allowing the hip of the kicking leg to open outwards can reduce the effectiveness and focus on the glutes.

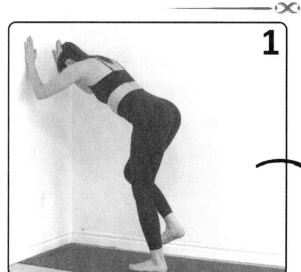

1

Stand with your feet hip-width apart, facing the wall, an arm's length away. Place your hands on the wall and hinge your hips back.

2

Keep your back stable and kick your right leg backwards and up. Slowly bring it back down (1) and repeat.

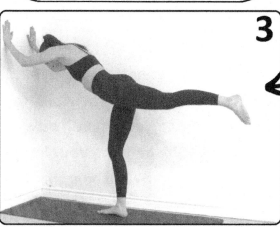

3

Do the same with the left leg , keep your back stable and kick your left leg backwards and up. Slowly bring it back down and repeat.

Wall Elevated Split Squat

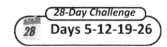
BENEFITS

- Strengthens the quadriceps, glutes, and hamstrings with a focus on one leg at a time for balanced muscle development.
- Enhances stability, balance, and core engagement.
- Improves hip flexibility and mobility.

TIPS

- Start by facing away from the wall, placing the rear foot on the wall at a comfortable height.
- Ensure your front foot is far enough forward to allow a deep squat without the knee passing the toes.
- Lower into the squat slowly, keeping the front knee aligned with the foot. Drive up through the heel of the front leg, maintaining a strong, engaged core for stability.
- Common Mistakes: Allowing the front knee to extend past the toes can lead to strain, and losing focus on core engagement may reduce stability and effectiveness of the exercise.

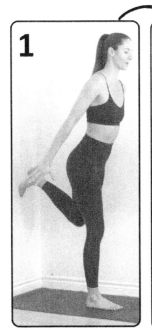
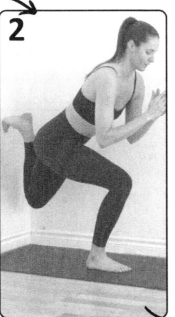
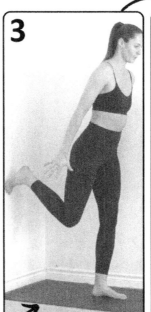
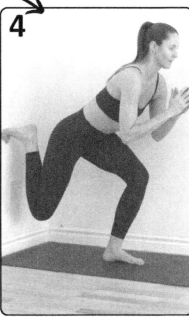

Stand hip-width apart facing away from the wall. Lift your left leg behind you and rest your foot on the wall. Hold this position and lower yourself down into a split squat by bending your right knee. Come back up by pushing through the heel of your right leg.

Stand hip-width apart facing away from the wall. Lift your right leg behind you and rest your foot on the wall. Hold this position and lower yourself down into a split squat by bending your left knee. Come back up by pushing through the heel of your left leg.

Wall Arm Angels

BENEFITS

- Improves shoulder mobility and upper back strength.
- Enhances postural awareness by activating the scapular stabilizers.
- Stretches the chest and front shoulder muscles.

TIPS

- Keep your lower back and arms in contact with the wall at all times.
- Move your arms slowly and deliberately to feel the muscles in your upper back working.
- Maintain a slight knee bend and core engagement for stability.
- Breathe smoothly as you slide your arms up and down the wall.
- Common Mistakes: Allowing the lower back to arch away from the wall or the arms to lift off the wall reduces the effectiveness of the exercise.

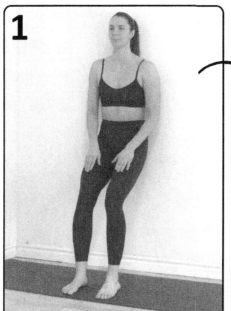

1 Stand with your back against a wall and your feet hip-width apart, slightly away from the wall. Bend your knees slightly and press your lower back into the wall.

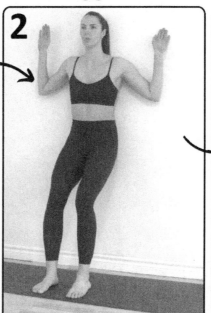

2 Bend your elbows at a 90-degree angle and rest the back of your arms on the wall.

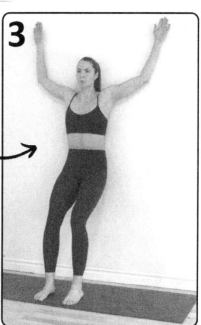

3 Activate your upper back and slide your arms up the wall as high as you can while maintaining contact with the wall. Slowly lower your arms back down (2) and repeat.

Wall Arm Butterflies

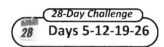

28-Day Challenge
Days 5-12-19-26

BENEFITS

- Strengthens the muscles of the upper back and shoulders.
- Encourages scapular retraction and promotes good posture.
- Stretches the pectoral muscles, beneficial for chest opening.

TIPS

- Keep your lower back pressed against the wall to maintain spinal alignment. Focus on squeezing the shoulder blades together as you open your arms.
- Keep elbows at shoulder height to maximize engagement of the upper back.
- Common Mistakes: Dropping the elbows below shoulder height can decrease the effectiveness, and not pressing the lower back into the wall can compromise posture.

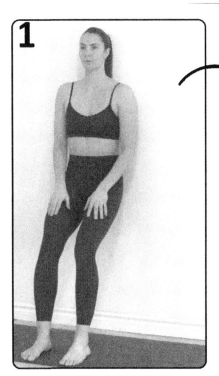

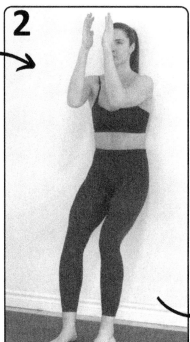

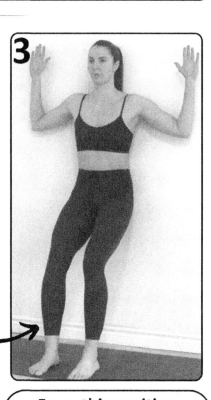

Stand with your back against a wall and your feet hip-width apart, slightly away from the wall.

Bend your elbows at a 90-degree angle and raise them to shoulder height. Bend your knees slightly.

From this position, squeeze your shoulder blades together and open your arms up all the way until your elbows touch the wall. Slowly return to the starting position (2) and repeat.

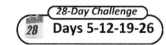
BENEFITS

- Deeply stretches the piriformis and gluteal muscles enhancing hip flexibility.
- Aids in relieving tension in the lower back and hips.
- Contributes to improved mobility.

TIPS

- Keep the foot of the non-crossed leg firmly against the wall to ensure stability and proper alignment.
- Use controlled breathing to relax deeper into the stretch, helping to release tension more effectively.
- Aim for symmetry in the stretch on both sides to maintain balanced flexibility and prevent muscular imbalances.
- Common Mistakes: Uneven pressure or alignment can lead to less effective stretching and potential discomfort.

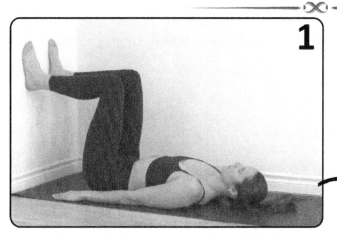

1

Lie on the ground with your feet on the wall and your knees bent at a 90-degree angle.

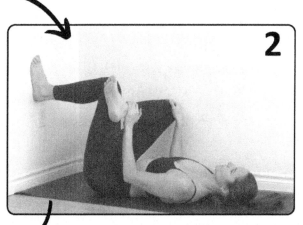

2

Place your left ankle on your right knee. Gently push your left thigh back, feeling a stretch in your left hip.

Place your right ankle on your left knee. Gently push your right thigh back, feeling a stretch in your right hip.

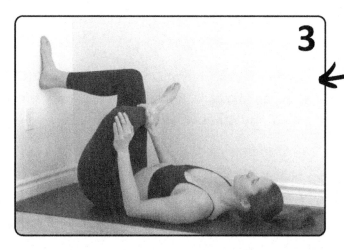

3

Days 6-13-20-27: Flexibility, Strength, and Balance

Welcome to Day 6 of your 28-day Wall Pilates journey! Today's routine is designed to enhance your flexibility, strength, and balance with a series of targeted exercises. Let's get started:

Warm-Up: Wall Hip Flexor Stretch

Begin your session with the _Wall Hip Flexor Stretch_, an essential movement to loosen up your hip flexors and improve your lower body mobility, setting a positive tone for the rest of your workout.

Core: Wall Elevated Plank Side Steps & Wall Standing Knee Drives

Activate your core with _Wall Elevated Plank Side Steps_, focusing on lateral movement to engage your obliques and stabilize your core.

Increase your heart rate and core engagement with _Wall Standing Knee Drives_. This dynamic movement not only targets your abdominals but also improves your **coordination and stamina**.

Lower Body: Wall Glute Kickbacks Pulses, Wall Glute Rainbow, Hip Adduction, Single Leg Bridge Leg Circles

Intensify your lower body workout with _Wall Glute Kickback Pulses_ and _Wall Glute Rainbow_ exercises, perfect for sculpting your glutes and thighs while enhancing your muscular endurance.

Hip Adduction and _Single Leg Bridge Leg Circles_ will focus on your inner thighs and glutes, promoting strength and flexibility. These exercises are crucial for a balanced lower body routine, ensuring all muscle groups are engaged.

Upper Body: Wall Triceps Press & Wall Side Bends

Strengthen your upper body with the _Wall Triceps Press_, targeting your triceps for toned arms and improved upper body strength.

Incorporate _Wall Side Bends_ to work on your obliques, enhancing your core strength and side-to-side flexibility, an essential aspect of a balanced fitness regimen.

Cool-Down: Hamstring Stretch

Conclude your workout with a _Hamstring Stretch_, a vital movement to relax and lengthen your hamstrings, reducing the risk of injury and promoting flexibility in your lower body.

Today's 10-minute routine is a comprehensive blend of exercises designed to work every major muscle group, with a special focus on improving flexibility, strength, and balance. Remember to spend **1 minute** on each exercise, adjusting the intensity as needed to match your fitness level.

Stay motivated and focused as you progress through Day 6, embracing each exercise as a step closer to achieving your health and wellness goals. Remember, the journey is as rewarding as the destination, so enjoy every moment of your Wall Pilates experience.

Wall Hip Flexor Stretch - Left

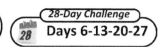
BENEFITS

- Stretches the hip flexors and quadriceps, key for hip mobility.
- Alleviates tightness in the front of the hip, which can benefit posture and lower back comfort.
- Assists in counteracting the effects of prolonged sitting.

TIPS

- Begin in the all-fours position and carefully place your knee and foot against the wall.
- Transition to an upright position smoothly, using the wall for balance.
- Lean back gently to intensify the stretch without straining.
- Keep your upper body straight and engage your glutes for a deeper stretch.
- Common Mistakes: Moving too quickly into the stretch or not engaging the glutes can lessen the stretch's effectiveness and potentially cause discomfort.

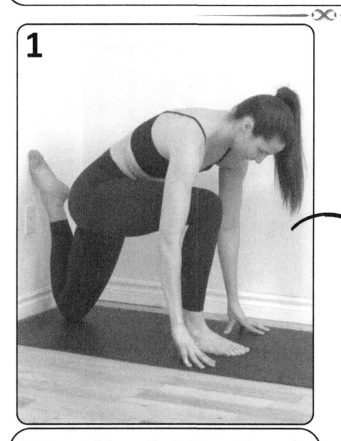

1

Start on all fours facing away from the wall. Lift your left knee up and place it as close to the wall as possible with the top of your foot resting on the wall.

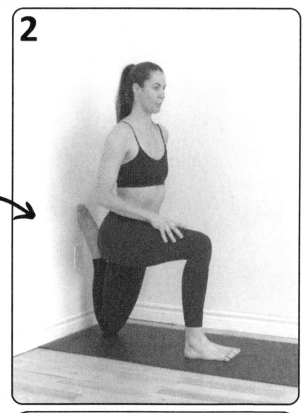

2

Lift your upper body up to come onto your right foot. Gently lean back towards the wall to feel a stretch in your left quadriceps and hip flexor.

Wall Hip Flexor Stretch - Right

 28-Day Challenge Days 6-13-20-27

BENEFITS

- Stretches the hip flexors and quadriceps, key for hip mobility.
- Alleviates tightness in the front of the hip, which can benefit posture and lower back comfort.
- Assists in counteracting the effects of prolonged sitting.

TIPS

- Begin in the all-fours position and carefully place your knee and foot against the wall.
- Transition to an upright position smoothly, using the wall for balance.
- Lean back gently to intensify the stretch without straining.
- Keep your upper body straight and engage your glutes for a deeper stretch.
- Common Mistakes: Moving too quickly into the stretch or not engaging the glutes can lessen the stretch's effectiveness and potentially cause discomfort.

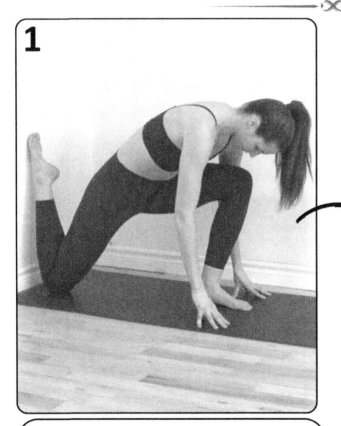

1 Start on all fours facing away from the wall. Lift your right knee up and place it as close to the wall as possible with the top of your foot resting on the wall.

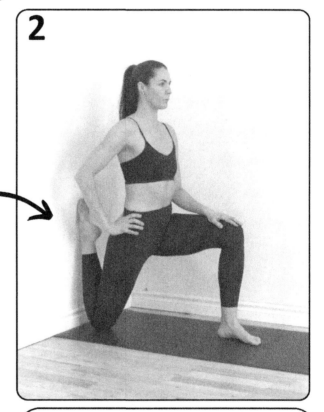

2 Lift your upper body up to come onto your left foot. Gently lean back towards the wall to feel a stretch in your right quadriceps and hip flexor.

Wall Elevated Plank Side Steps

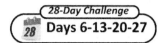
28-Day Challenge
Days 6-13-20-27

BENEFITS

- Enhances lateral core stability and strength.
- Engages and strengthens the shoulder muscles.
- Improves coordination and balance.

TIPS

- Maintain a strong, engaged core throughout to support your spine.
- Ensure your wrists stay directly under your shoulders for stability.
- Move each foot sideways in a measured manner to maintain form.
- Common Mistakes: Shifting the hips too much during the steps can reduce core engagement. Ensure minimal hip sway for maximum effectiveness.

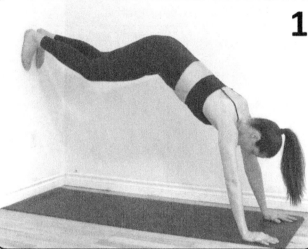

1

Start on all fours facing away from the wall. Place your feet on the wall, holding an elevated high plank with your wrists under your shoulders and your core engaged.

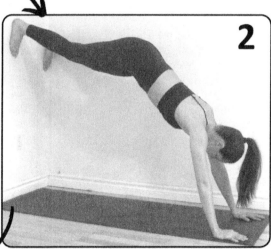

2

From this position, step sideways with your left foot.

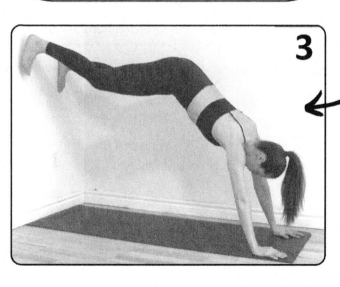

3

Bring it back to its starting position (1) and repeat with your right foot.

Wall Standing Knee Drives

BENEFITS

- Strengthens the core, especially the lower abdominals.
- Improves balance and lower body coordination.
- Activates the hip flexors.

TIPS

- Press your lower back firmly against the wall for stability and support.
- Engage your core throughout the exercise to maximize the benefits and protect your spine.
- Lift each knee as high as comfortably possible, focusing on controlled movements.
- Keep the pace steady, ensuring quality of movement over speed.
- Common Mistakes: Not engaging the core fully or jerking the knee up too quickly can reduce effectiveness.

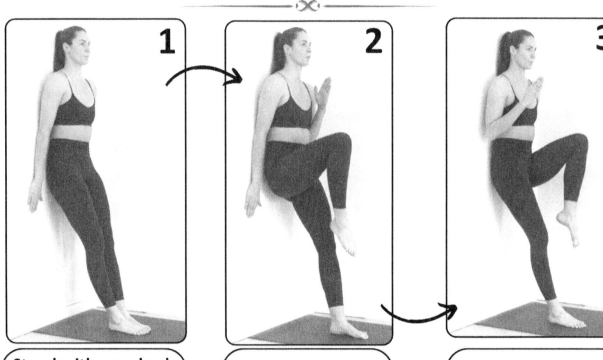

1 Stand with your back against the wall and your feet hip-width apart, slightly away from the wall. Keep your core engaged and lower back pressed into the wall.

2 From this position, drive your right knee up towards your chest.

3 Lower it back down and repeat with the left knee. Continue alternating legs each time.

Wall Glute Kickbacks Pulses

BENEFITS

- Intensifies the glute engagement compared to standard kickbacks.
- Increases muscle endurance and strength in the glutes.
- Enhances stability and balance

TIPS

- Avoid arching your back to focus the work on your glutes.
- Keep the standing leg slightly bent for stability and safety.
- Use your hands against the wall to maintain balance and allow for greater focus on the glute muscles.
- Common Mistakes: Losing the raised leg's height during pulses or allowing the hips to rotate can diminish the exercise's effectiveness.

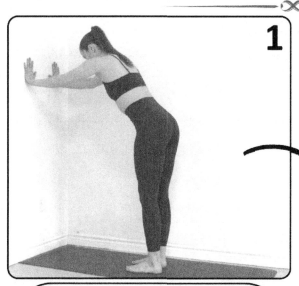

1

Stand with your feet hip-width apart, facing the wall, an arm's length away. Place your hands on the wall and hinge your hips back.

Keep your back stable and kick your right leg backwards and up. From this position, perform small pulses with your right leg.

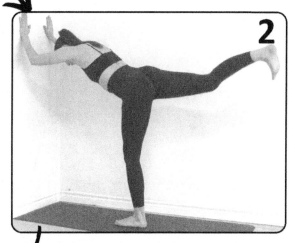

2

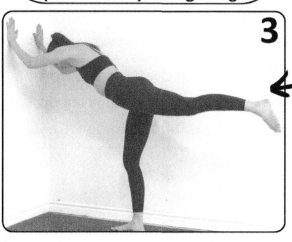

3

Do the same with the left leg , kick your left leg backwards and up. From this position, perform small pulses with your left leg.

81

Wall Glute Rainbow- Right

BENEFITS

- Enhances gluteus maximus engagement while also targeting the gluteus medius for a rounded workout.
- Improves hip mobility and stability.
- Promotes coordination and balance through controlled movement.

TIPS

- Focus on creating a wide, controlled arc with your right leg to fully engage the glutes.
- Keep your core engaged and your back stable to support the movement and protect your spine.
- Use your hands against the wall for balance, allowing you to concentrate on the leg movement.
- Aim for a smooth, controlled motion, ensuring the leg movement is driven by your glutes.
- Common Mistakes: Rushing the movement or not maintaining a stable core can lead to reduced effectiveness and potential strain.

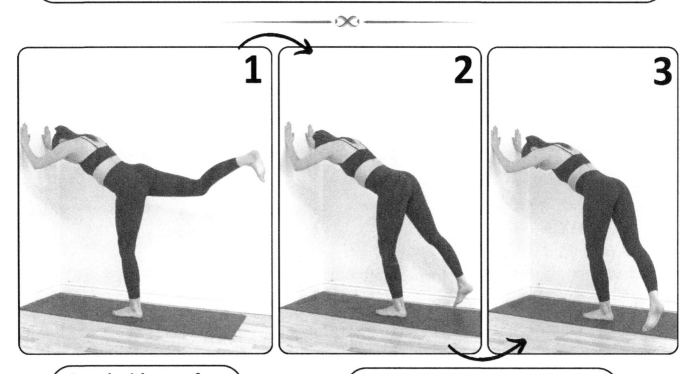

Stand with your feet hip-width apart, facing the wall, an arm's length away. Place your hands on the wall and hinge your hips back.

Keep your back stable and core engaged. Kick your right leg up, creating a rainbow shape with it.

Wall Glute Rainbow - Left

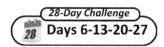
28-Day Challenge
Days 6-13-20-27

BENEFITS

- Targets and strengthens the left gluteus maximus and medius for comprehensive lower body toning.
- Increases hip mobility and enhances lateral movement control.
- Strengthens core stability and balance with unilateral movement.

TIPS

- Engage your core and maintain a flat back to provide stability during the exercise.
- Create a wide, controlled arc with your left leg, focusing on engaging the glute muscles.
- Use the wall for steady support, allowing greater concentration on the leg movement.
- Execute the movement smoothly, ensuring it is driven by glute activation.
- Common Mistakes: Failing to keep the core engaged or allowing the hips to rotate can diminish the exercise's effectiveness and risk lower back strain.

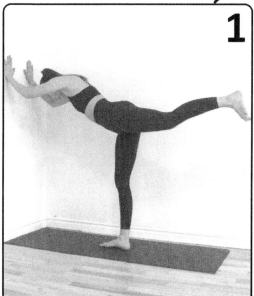

1

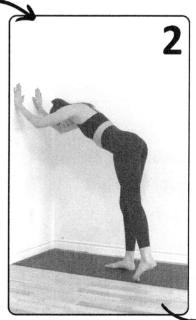

2

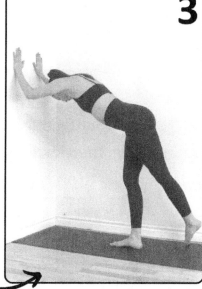

3

Stand with your feet hip-width apart, facing the wall, an arm's length away. Place your hands on the wall and hinge your hips back.

Keep your back stable and core engaged. Kick your left leg up, creating a rainbow shape with it.

Hip Adduction

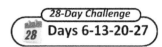

28-Day Challenge
Days 6-13-20-27

BENEFITS

- Targets and strengthens the adductor muscles (inner thighs) on both sides.
- Improves hip stability and mobility.
- Helps correct muscular imbalances in the lower body.

TIPS

- Ensure smooth, controlled movements to maintain the exercise's effectiveness and safety. Alternate sides to work both sets of adductor muscles evenly.
- Common Mistakes: Allowing the body to roll forward or back reduces the effectiveness of the adduction and can lead to strain. Keep movements controlled and focused to ensure the inner thighs are properly targeted.

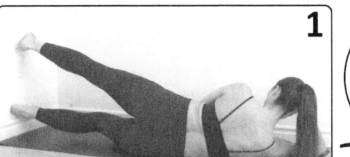

1

Lie on the ground on your right side with your head resting in your hand. Keep your legs straight. Place your left foot on the wall.

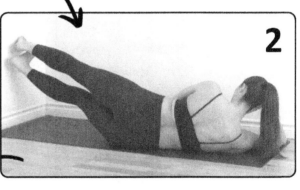

2

Lift your right leg to meet your left leg, then lower it back down in a controlled manner.

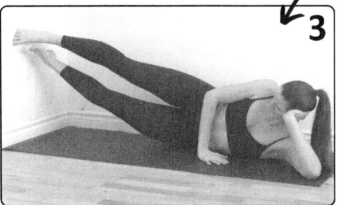

3

Lie on the ground on your left side with your head resting in your hand. Keep your legs straight. Place your right foot on the wall. Lift your left leg to meet your right leg, then lower it back down in a controlled manner.

Single Leg Bridge Leg Circles

BENEFITS

- Strengthens the glutes, hamstrings, and core.
- Enhances hip mobility and stability through controlled leg movements.
- Improves coordination and balance.

TIPS

- Ensure a strong glute bridge position with one leg before starting the circles to maintain stability. Keep the extended leg's movements small and controlled, focusing on the mobility of the hip joint.
- Perform the leg circles smoothly.
- Switch legs to ensure balanced strength and flexibility development.
- Common Mistakes: Dropping the hips during the circles or losing control of the movement can reduce the exercise's effectiveness and increase the risk of strain.

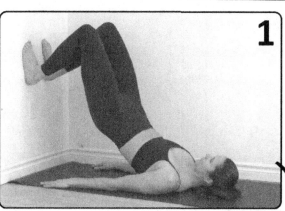

1

Lie on the ground with your feet on the wall. Keep your knees bent at a 90-degree angle. Push through your heels to lift your hips up, squeezing your glutes at the top of this movement.

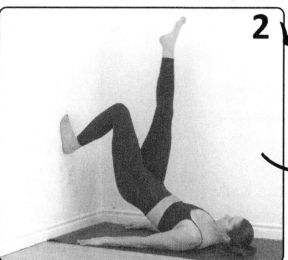

2

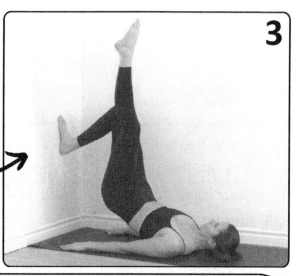

3

Extend your right leg and perform small circles with your foot while keeping everything else steady. At the end of the exercise, place your right foot back on the wall (1) and lower your hips back down in a controlled manner. Repeat the exercise, switching the positions of your legs (3).

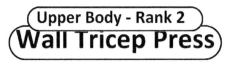

BENEFITS
- Specifically targets and strengthens the triceps.
- Helps improve upper body muscle tone and definition.
- Can enhance overall arm strength and stability.

TIPS
- Keep your elbows close to your body to focus the work on your triceps. Engage your core and maintain a straight back to support proper form.
- Lower yourself until your elbows gently touch the wall, then press back up powerfully. Distribute your weight evenly through your feet and palms for balance.
- Common Mistakes: Allowing your elbows to flare out can shift the focus away from the triceps.

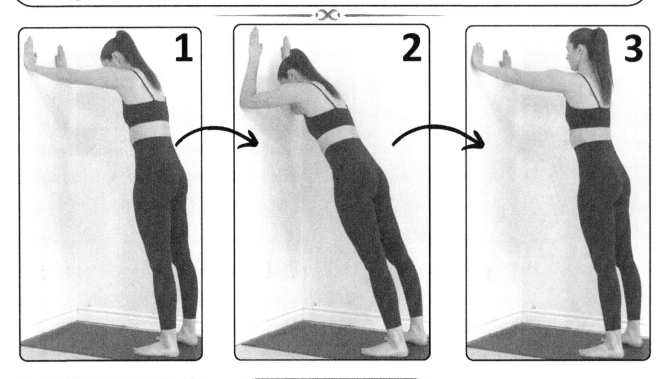

Stand facing the wall with your feet hip-width apart. Place your hands on the wall, slightly wider than shoulder width. Maintain this position by keeping your core engaged and back straight.

From there, lower yourself until your elbows touch the wall.

Push through the palms of your hands to push yourself back up, activating your triceps as you come up.

Wall Side Bends

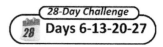

BENEFITS

- Stretches and strengthens the oblique muscles on both sides of the torso.
- Enhances spinal mobility and flexibility.
- Can help alleviate tightness in the lateral sides of the body.

TIPS

- As you bend, focus on keeping your hips stable and aligned, avoiding any forward or backward tilting. Extend the opposite arm over your head to deepen the stretch along the side body.
- Gently touch the wall with your extended hand, using it as a guide to ensure a full side bend.
- Return to the starting position with control, engaging your core to lift your torso back up.
- Common Mistakes: Bending too far or too quickly can strain the muscles. Ensure the movement is controlled and within a comfortable range of motion to maximize benefits and safety.

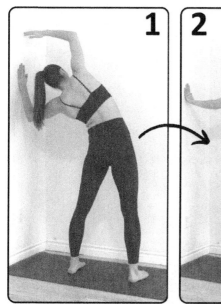
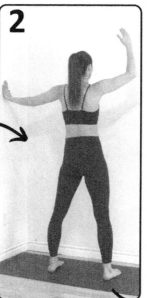
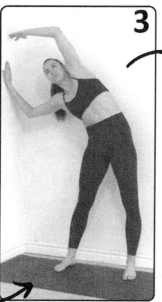
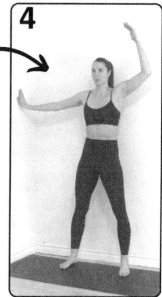

Stand with your feet shoulder-width apart next to the wall. Place your left hand on the wall. Bend towards your left side while lifting your right arm up and over your head. Touch the wall with your right hand and return to the starting position.

Stand with your feet shoulder-width apart next to the wall. Place your right hand on the wall. Bend towards your right side while lifting your left arm up and over your head. Touch the wall with your left hand and return to the starting position.

Hamstring Stretch

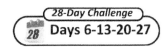

BENEFITS

- Effectively stretches the hamstrings, promoting flexibility and reducing tightness.
- Aids in relieving tension in the lower back and legs.
- Enhances circulation to the lower extremities.

TIPS

- Gently pull one leg towards you while keeping the other leg straight and pressed against the wall.
- Use your hands to guide the stretch, keeping the foot of the stretching leg flexed to also target the calf. Maintain a steady, even breath to help deepen the stretch without forcing.
- Common Mistakes: Pulling the leg too forcefully can strain the muscles, and allowing the opposite leg to bend or come off the wall reduces the effectiveness of the stretch.

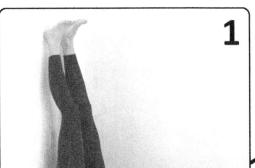

1

Lie on the ground with your legs up the wall. Keep your legs straight.

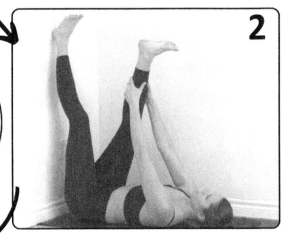

2

Bring your right leg off the wall and, using your hands, gently pull your leg towards you to stretch your right hamstring. Keep your foot flexed to feel a stretch in your right calf.

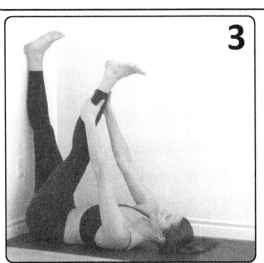

3

Bring your left leg off the wall and, using your hands, gently pull your leg towards you to stretch your left hamstring. Keep your foot flexed to feel a stretch in your left calf.

Days 7-14-21-28: Integration and Harmony

Day 7 marks the end of your first week on this **28-Day Wall Pilates** path. Today's practice aims to integrate the work of the past days into a harmonious session that challenges and nurtures your body.

Warm-Up: Standing Wall Hip Circles

Kickstart your session with _Standing Wall Hip Circles_ to loosen your hips and lower body, setting a dynamic tone for today's workout. It's a fantastic way to awaken your muscles and joints.

Core: Wall Pilates 100's & Double Leg Stretch

Elevate your core strength with the _Wall Pilates 100's_, an exercise that stimulates deep abdominal engagement and enhances breath control, key to core stability and power.

The _Double Leg Stretch_ further challenges your core, focusing on abdominal endurance and flexibility, essential for a strong, balanced core.

Lower Body: Wall Reverse Lunges, Wall Diamonds, Glute Bridge Pulses, Wall Laying Hip Adductions

Strengthen your lower body with _Wall Reverse Lunges_ and _Wall Diamonds_, which sculpt your legs and glutes while improving your balance and functional movement.

Glute Bridge Pulses and _Wall Laying Hip Adductions_ emphasize your glutes and inner thighs, promoting muscle tone and endurance with movements that support pelvic health and stability.

Upper Body: Wall Commando Planks & Wall Pike

Wall Commando Planks will test your upper body strength and core stability, transitioning between different levels of plank positions to engage your shoulders, chest, and arms.

The _Wall Pike_ shifts focus to your shoulders and back, enhancing upper body strength and flexibility, vital for a comprehensive Pilates practice.

Cool-Down: Leg Swings

Conclude with _Leg Swings_ to relax and stretch your legs, hips, and lower back, ensuring your body recovers properly and remains flexible, a perfect end to your weekly routine.

The final day of your weekly routine is a balanced mix of exercises designed to refine the strength, flexibility, and balance you've been working on. Each movement, lasting **1 minute**, brings you closer to your goals, offering a total of **10 minutes of focused**, effective Wall Pilates practice.

Embrace the achievements of your first week, acknowledging the progress and dedication you've shown. As you continue on this journey, remember that each day is an opportunity to grow stronger, more flexible, and in greater harmony with your body's needs.

Standing Wall Hip Circles - Left

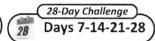
BENEFITS

- Enhances hip mobility and flexibility.
- Strengthens the standing leg's stability and balance.
- Activates the hip joint's range of motion.

TIPS

- Use the wall for steady support and maintain a slight bend in your standing knee.
- Focus on controlled, smooth circles to engage the hip muscles fully.
- Start with small circles, gradually increasing the size as flexibility improves.
- Perform equal numbers of circles in both directions for balance.
- Common Mistakes: Rushing the circles can lead to less control, and locking the standing knee may reduce stability.

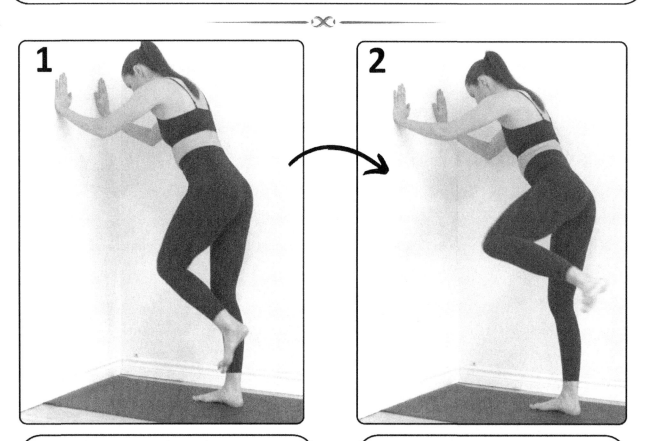

1 Stand facing a wall with your hands placed on the wall at shoulder height for balance. Stand on your right foot, maintaining a slight bend in the knee.

2 Lift your left leg, bending at the knee, and bring your knee up to hip level. Begin to draw circles in the air with your lifted knee.

Standing Wall Hip Circles - Right

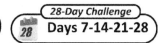

28-Day Challenge
Days 7-14-21-28

BENEFITS

- Enhances hip mobility and flexibility.
- Strengthens the standing leg's stability and balance.
- Activates the hip joint's range of motion.

TIPS

- Use the wall for steady support and maintain a slight bend in your standing knee.
- Focus on controlled, smooth circles to engage the hip muscles fully.
- Start with small circles, gradually increasing the size as flexibility improves.
- Perform equal numbers of circles in both directions for balance.
- Common Mistakes: Rushing the circles can lead to less control, and locking the standing knee may reduce stability.

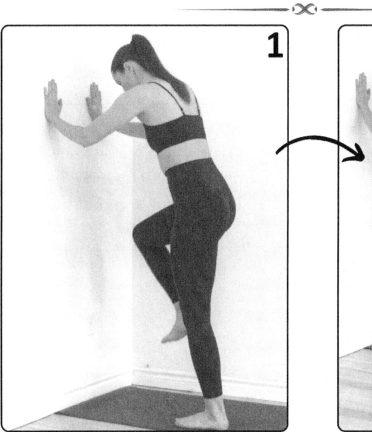

1

Stand facing a wall with your hands placed on the wall at shoulder height for balance. Stand on your left foot, keeping a slight bend in the knee.

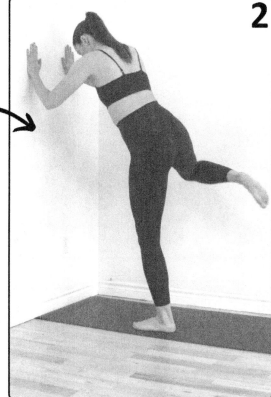

2

Lift your right leg, bending at the knee, and bring your knee up to hip level. Begin to draw circles in the air with your lifted knee.

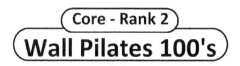

Core - Rank 2
Wall Pilates 100's

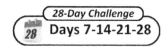

28-Day Challenge
Days 7-14-21-28

BENEFITS

- Enhances core strength and endurance.
- Promotes deep abdominal engagement.
- Improves breathing control and coordination.

TIPS

- Focus on stabilizing your core to keep your back and legs steady.
- Perform small, controlled arm pulses, engaging your shoulder muscles.
- Use rhythmic breathing, inhaling for five pulses and exhaling for five, to complement the movement.
- Keep your gaze forward and chin slightly tucked to maintain a neutral neck.
- Common Mistakes: Losing core engagement can compromise the exercise's effectiveness. Ensure your movements are precise and controlled to avoid straining your neck or lower back.

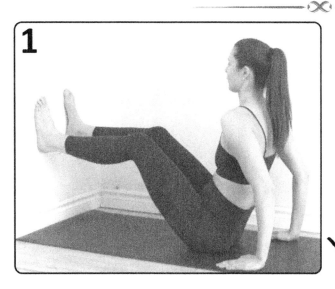

Start in a seated position with your knees bent at a 45-degree angle, facing the wall. Shift your weight onto your sit bones and bring your feet up onto the wall. Extend your arms out to your sides.

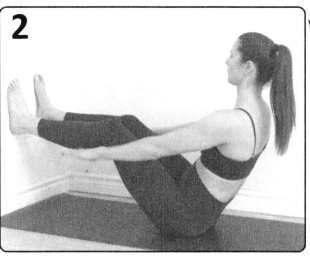

From this position, perform small pulses with your hands while keeping everything else stable.

Double Leg Stretch

BENEFITS

- Strengthens the core, particularly the deep abdominal muscles.
- Enhances coordination and flexibility in the legs.
- Improves pelvic stability and control.

TIPS

- Start with your legs gently bent to avoid straining the lower back.
- As you bring your knees in, focus on engaging the abdominals to deepen the core work. Use your arms to gently hug your legs, enhancing the stretch without forcing the movement.
- Common Mistakes: Extending the legs too quickly can lead to lower back arching. Ensure your movements are controlled and your back remains pressed to the ground.

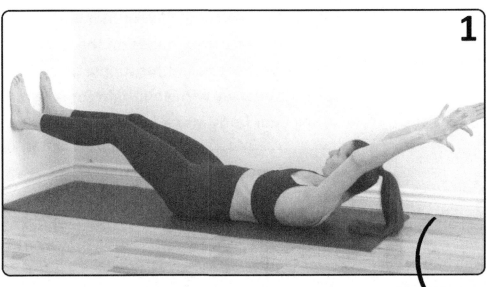

1 Lie on the ground on your back with your feet on the wall. Keep your legs straight with a gentle bend in your knees. Extend your arms behind you.

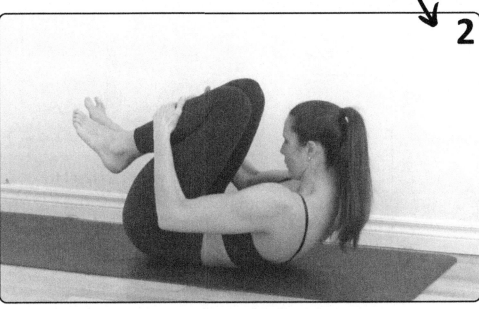

2 Bend both knees and bring the knees in towards your chest. Use your arms to hug the legs in. Hold briefly, then release the legs and extend the arms (1).

Wall Reverse Lunges

BENEFITS

- Strengthens the glutes, quadriceps, and hamstrings.
- Enhances lower body stability and balance.
- Improves hip mobility and knee alignment.

TIPS

- Keep your front knee aligned over your ankle to protect the joint.
- Lower into the lunge with control, keeping the movement smooth.
- Drive through the heel of your front foot to return to the starting position, engaging your glutes.
- Common Mistakes: Not maintaining a 90-degree angle in both knees can reduce the effectiveness of the lunge.

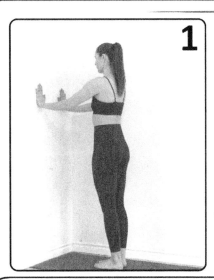

1

Stand facing a wall, with your feet hip-width apart. Place your hands on the wall at about chest height for support.
Take a step back with your right foot, lowering your body into a lunge position.

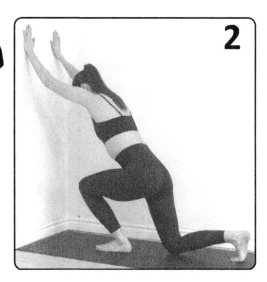

2

Both knees should be bent at a 90-degree angle. Ensure that your left knee remains directly above your left ankle and your right knee hovers slightly above the floor.

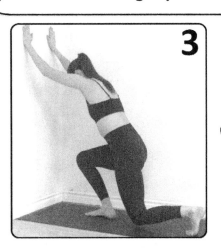

3

Push through your left heel to return to the starting position (1). Repeat the lunge with your left foot stepping back.

Wall Diamonds

BENEFITS

- Enhances flexibility and mobility in the hips and inner thighs.
- Promotes relaxation in the lower back and pelvic area.
- Can help alleviate tightness in the groin and improve leg movement range.

TIPS

- Allow your knees to gently fall to the sides, opening up the hips without forcing them.
- Slide your feet down the wall smoothly, keeping the soles pressed together to maintain the diamond shape.
- Go as low as comfortable, focusing on the stretch.
- Use your hands for gentle support on your knees or thighs if needed to encourage relaxation.
- Common Mistakes: Pushing the knees or feet too aggressively can lead to strain. Listen to your body and stretch to the point of mild tension, not pain.

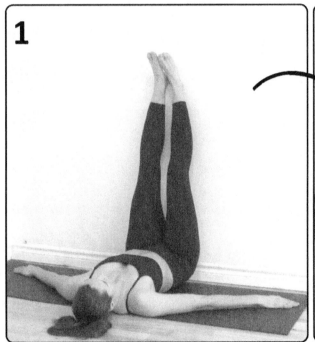

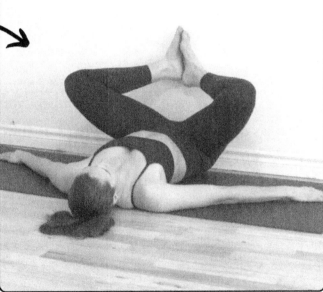

Lie on the ground with your legs up against the wall. Let your knees drop and press the soles of your feet together.

From this position, slide your feet down the wall, creating a diamond shape with your legs. Go as low as you can, then slide your legs back up the wall (1).

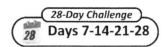

BENEFITS

- Intensifies glute engagement and strengthens the muscles.
- Enhances hip mobility and stability.
- Improves lower back support and core strength.

TIPS

- Keep your feet against the wall and your knees bent to maintain form.
- Focus on lifting your hips using your glutes, not your lower back.
- Perform controlled pulses at the top of the bridge to maximize muscle activation. Ensure your movements are steady and rhythmic to maintain continuous tension on the glutes.
- Common Mistakes: Allowing the hips to drop between pulses or using momentum rather than muscle control can reduce the effectiveness.

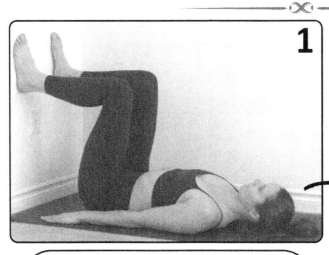

1

Lie on the ground with your feet on the wall. Keep your knees bent at a 90-degree angle.

2

Push through your heels to lift your hips up, squeezing your glutes at the top of this movement. While in this elevated position, perform small pulses with your hips.

3

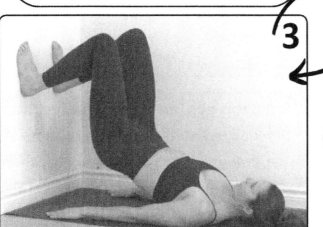

At the end of the exercise, slowly lower your hips back down (1).

(Lower Body - Rank 1)

Wall Lying Hip Adductions

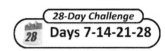

28-Day Challenge
Days 7-14-21-28

BENEFITS

- Strengthens the inner thigh muscles (adductors).
- Improves hip mobility and flexibility.
- Can aid in preventing groin injuries and improving lower body alignment.

TIPS

- Start with your legs straight up against the wall, then slide them out to a comfortable split position. Focus on using your inner thigh muscles to draw your legs back together.
- Keep the movement controlled and smooth, ensuring even engagement on both sides.
- Adjust the range of motion according to your flexibility level.
- Common Mistakes: Overstretching or forcing the legs too far apart can lead to strain. Listen to your body and avoid pushing beyond a comfortable stretch.

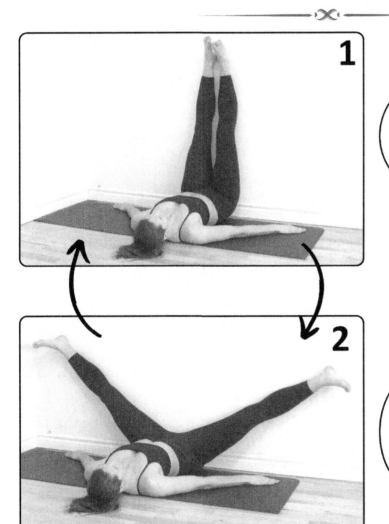

1

Lie on the ground with your legs up the wall. Slide your feet out as if you were performing a split.

2

Go as far as you can go, then using your inner thighs, pull your legs back up to the starting position.

Wall Commando Planks

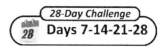
BENEFITS

- Enhances core stability and strength.
- Improves shoulder endurance and coordination.
- Challenges the body with dynamic movement and stability control.

TIPS

- Maintain a strong, engaged core to protect the spine and increase effectiveness.
- Transition smoothly between hand and elbow positions to keep tension on the core and shoulders.
- Alternate the leading arm to promote balanced strength and coordination. Keep the back straight and avoid hip sagging or piking throughout the exercise.
- Common Mistakes: Rushing the movements can lead to a loss of form, and not alternating the leading arm may result in uneven muscle development.

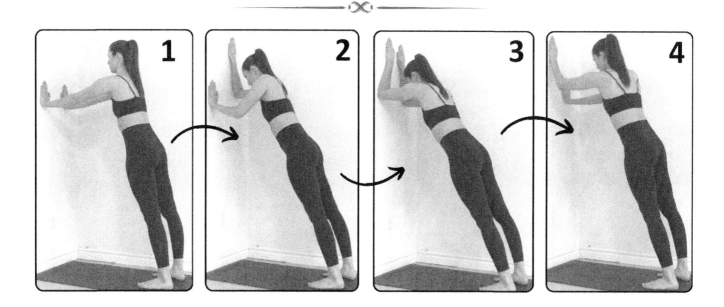

Stand facing the wall with your feet hip-width apart. Place your hands on the wall at shoulder level.

Bend your right elbow and place it onto the wall (2), then repeat with your left elbow (3). Now reverse the movement, coming back into the starting position (1).

Repeat, this time leading with the left elbow.

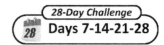
BENEFITS

- Strengthens the shoulders, upper back, and core.
- Increases hamstring flexibility and hip mobility.
- Enhances body control and stability.

TIPS

- Start with shins against the wall and elbows under shoulders for support. Lift hips smoothly, pressing heels towards the wall to deepen the stretch.
- Keep the core tight to support the movement and protect the lower back.
- Move in and out of the pike position with controlled, deliberate motions.
- Common Mistakes: Collapsing the back during the pike or not engaging the core can reduce the effectiveness of the exercise and risk injury.

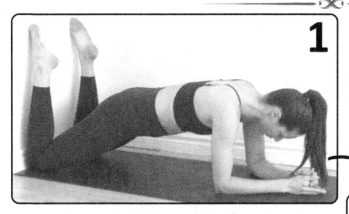

1

Start on your stomach with knees bent at a 90-degree angle and your shins pressed against the wall. Come up onto your elbows.

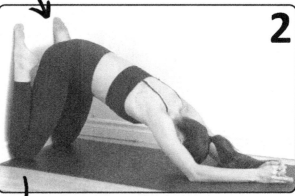

2

From here, push your hips up and back to make contact with your feet.

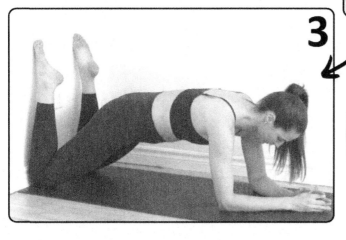

3

Slowly return to the starting position, keeping your core engaged the entire time. Continue, gently moving between the two positions.

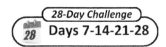
BENEFITS

- Enhances dynamic flexibility in the hips and legs.
- Prepares muscles and joints for exercise by increasing blood flow.
- Improves range of motion and mobility.

TIPS

- Use the wall for balance, lightly placing your hand to stabilize your body. Allow your leg to swing freely front to back, gradually increasing the range as you warm up.
- Keep your torso upright and engage your core to maintain stability.
- Focus on a fluid motion, avoiding any jerky movements.
- Alternate legs to ensure balanced flexibility and mobility.
- Common Mistakes: Swinging the leg too forcefully from the start can lead to muscle strain. Begin gently and gradually increase the swing's amplitude.

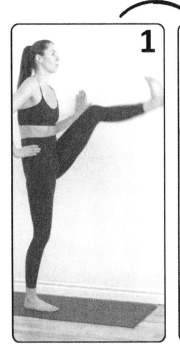

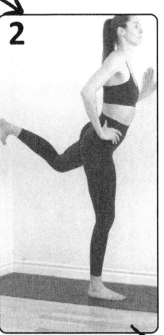

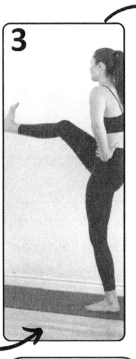

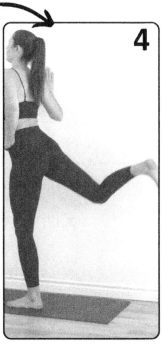

1 Stand with your feet hip-width apart next to a wall. Place your left hand on the wall for support.

2 Swing your left leg front to back, using momentum to increase your range of motion.

3 Stand with your feet hip-width apart next to a wall. Place your right hand on the wall for support.

4 Swing your right leg front to back, using momentum to increase your range of motion.

Tailored Strength: Wall Pilates for Women's Unique Needs

Embracing Women's Health Journeys

I'm not just stopping with the 28-Day Challenge Program. Following this transformative journey, I'm excited to introduce a special section dedicated to addressing women's health issues through the lens of Wall Pilates. This segment is meticulously crafted to offer bonus exercises that specifically target health concerns prevalent among women, such as menstrual pain, menopause disorders, and post-pregnancy form recovery.

I recognize the unique challenges and changes a woman's body goes through at different stages of life. Therefore, this section aims to provide supportive, therapeutic exercises designed to alleviate discomfort, enhance well-being, and promote healing. Together, we'll explore these targeted exercises, empowering you to take control of your well-being and live a life of balance, strength, and vitality. Feel free to integrate these exercises with your daily workout routine.

Nurturing Pelvic Floor Health

The pelvic floor is a critical area for women, supporting vital functions and contributing to overall well-being. Life's milestones, such as childbirth and aging, can challenge these muscles, leading to discomfort and other concerns. Wall Pilates steps in with targeted exercises that help strengthen and rejuvenate the pelvic floor, promoting a sense of control and confidence, making it an ideal choice for women at any life stage, including those preparing for or recovering from childbirth, and those experiencing the hormonal changes of menopause.

The use of the wall as a prop provides stability and guidance, ensuring exercises are performed with proper alignment and focus, directly benefiting the pelvic floor. The practice emphasizes mindful movement and breathwork, integral components that enhance the connection to the pelvic floor. By coordinating breath with movement, each session becomes an opportunity to engage these muscles effectively, supporting their health and function.

Strengthening surrounding areas such as the core, glutes, and thighs, also plays a significant role in supporting pelvic floor health. Exercises like wall squats and leg lifts not only target these supportive muscle groups but also encourage pelvic floor engagement, offering comprehensive benefits.

For women gradually returning to physical activity, Wall Pilates offers a customizable approach, allowing for a tailored pace that respects the body's healing process. Starting with basic stretches and progressively incorporating strength-focused exercises fosters a safe and effective recovery.

Beyond physical benefits, Wall Pilates contributes to stress reduction and mental well-being. The focus on breath and movement provides a calming effect, helping to alleviate tension, which can benefit the pelvic floor by reducing involuntary tightening.

Wall Pilates for Menstrual Discomfort

During menstruation, it's not uncommon to experience a range of discomforts. Wall Pilates exercises can offer gentle support, helping to ease tension and promote well-being without overexerting the body.

- **Wall Butterfly Stretch**: Opens hips, potentially alleviating cramps.

- **Seated Forward Folds:** the relaxation and gentle stretching of the lower back and pelvic area during this exercise may offer some relief from the discomfort associated with menstrual cramps by promoting relaxation and improving circulation.

- **Piriformis Stretch**: For some women, menstrual discomfort includes lower back and hip pain, partly due to muscular tension or imbalances. Regularly performing the Piriformis Stretch may help alleviate some of this discomfort by improving flexibility and reducing pressure on the pelvic area.

Wall Pilates After Pregnancy

Once your bundle of joy has arrived, the postpartum period is all about healing and finding your strength again. Wall Pilates is there to support you through this recovery, with exercises that gently ease you back into being active. It's all about rebuilding that core strength and taking care of the pelvic floor, which really goes through a lot during pregnancy and childbirth.

- **Wall Elevated Split Squat:** Strengthens lower body, helps regain stability and form.

- **Wall Hip Adduction:** Strengthens inner thighs, supports pelvic floor recovery.

- **Wall Single Leg Bridge Leg Circles:** Strengthens glutes and core, enhances pelvic stability.

- **Wall Single Leg Stretch**: Gently engages core, promotes post-pregnancy abdominal recovery.

- **Wall Supported Ankle Rolls:** After pregnancy, women may experience swelling or changes in their feet and ankles due to weight gain and fluid retention. This exercise can aid in restoring ankle mobility and reducing swelling, contributing to overall post-pregnancy recovery.

- **Wall Calf Raises:** Improves lower leg strength and stability, vital for balance and locomotion activities.

- **Clamshells:** They target the pelvic floor and hip stabilizers, muscles that are often weakened during pregnancy and childbirth. Strengthening these areas can help new mothers regain core stability, reduce the risk of incontinence, and improve posture, aiding in overall recovery.

Remember, checking in with your healthcare provider before jumping back into any exercise.

Wall Pilates During Menopause

Menopause brings its unique set of challenges, but Wall Pilates remains a gentle yet effective way to manage symptoms, focusing on exercises that promote strength, flexibility, and hormonal balance.

- **Wall Hamstring Stretch**: Addresses muscle tightness and improves flexibility, which can be beneficial during menopause.

- **Wall Seated Forward Folds**: Promotes overall relaxation, aiding in managing stress associated with menopause.

- **Seated Thoracic Rotations**: This exercise can help improve upper body flexibility and reduce stiffness, which can be beneficial during menopause when women might experience increased tension in the upper back and shoulders.

- **Wall Supported Ankle Rolls**: Helpful for improving circulation and reducing swelling, a common issue during menopause due to hormonal changes.

- **Wall Cobra Push Up**: Can assist in strengthening the back muscles, improving posture, and alleviating back pain, which is crucial as hormonal fluctuations during menopause can weaken bones and muscles.

- **Wall Squats**: This exercise strengthens the lower body, maintaining bone density and combating osteoporosis, a significant concern for menopausal women.

- **Wall Cat Cow**: Offers gentle spinal flexion and extension, promoting back flexibility and reducing stress, a common symptom during menopause.

- **Wall Plié Squats**: Strengthens the pelvic floor, thighs, and glutes, areas that can weaken during menopause, and supports hormonal balance through lower body strengthening.

- **Wall Standing Child's Pose**: This stretch can provide a sense of relaxation and relief from stress, helping to manage hot flashes and improve sleep quality.

- **Piriformis Stretch**: Useful for alleviating sciatic pain and discomfort in the buttocks and hips, which can be problematic due to hormonal changes affecting joints and muscles.

- **Butterfly Stretch**: Helps in maintaining hip flexibility and reducing tightness, promoting better circulation and relaxation.

For Reducing Tension and Headaches

Maintaining spinal health and reducing neck tension are key to managing headaches. The gentle movement of Wall Cat Cow, combined with the focused neck rotations, can significantly alleviate tension in the upper body, a common contributor to both tension headaches and overall stress.

- **Wall Cat Cow**: Soothes back and neck, promoting spinal health and flexibility.

- **Wall Side to Side Neck Rotations**: Eases neck stiffness, potentially reducing tension headaches.

- **Side Leg Swings:** By focusing on hip mobility, these swings can decrease stiffness and improve relaxation, potentially alleviating physical contributors to tension headaches.

- **Wall Toe Touch Crunches:** Helps alleviate tension throughout the body by promoting relaxation and stress relief. Strengthening the core also supports better posture, which can reduce physical stress and strain contributing to tension.

- **Single Leg Stretch:** Reduce overall body tension. By improving core strength and flexibility, the exercise can support better posture and reduce the physical stress that often contributes to tension.

- **Wall Side Bends**: help release muscular tension that often contributes to overall body stress and tension headaches.

- **Wall Double Leg Stretch**: Focuses on deep core engagement, supports back and pelvic health.

- **Piriformis Stretch**: Relieves buttock and back discomfort, useful for sedentary lifestyles or sciatic issues.

Some of the exercises I mentioned in this chapter have already been shown in the **28-Day Challenge**. In the following pages, I will cover the others.

Feel free to integrate these exercises into your daily routine!

Wall Calf Raises

BENEFITS

- Strengthens the calf muscles (gastrocnemius and soleus).
- Improves ankle stability and mobility.
- Enhances balance and supports posture.

TIPS

- Push evenly through the balls of both feet to lift your heels as high as possible.
- Hold the top position briefly to maximize calf muscle engagement.
- Lower your heels slowly to increase the stretch and strength training effect.
- Common Mistakes: Rushing the movement can reduce its effectiveness, and failing to fully extend the ankles may limit the development of strength and flexibility.

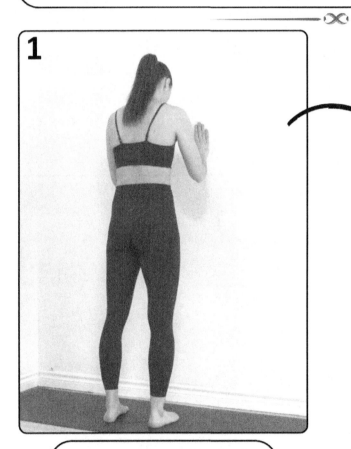

1

Stand facing a wall with your feet hip-width apart. Place your hands on the wall at about chest height for support.

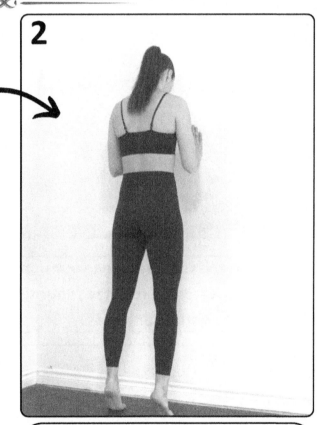

2

Raise your heels off the ground by pushing through the balls of your feet. Hold the raised position for a brief moment.
Lower your heels back down to the starting position and repeat.

Seated Forward Folds

BENEFITS

- Stretches the hamstrings and lower back, promoting flexibility and reducing tightness.
- Can alleviate tension in the upper body.
- Enhances circulation by encouraging a forward bend.

TIPS

- Extend your arms overhead to lengthen the spine before folding forward. Reach towards your feet with both hands, maintaining a flat back as much as possible.
- If you can't reach your feet, hold onto your shins or knees and gradually work on increasing your flexibility.
- Common Mistakes: Overstretching or forcing the torso towards the legs can lead to strain. Keep the fold gentle and within your comfortable range of motion.

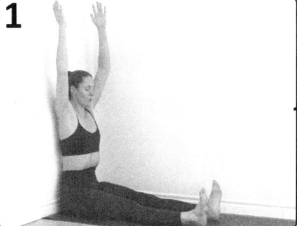

1

Start in a seated position with your back against the wall and your legs extended. Extend your arms above your head.

2

Bend at the torso to bring your upper body forward and reach for your feet with your hands.

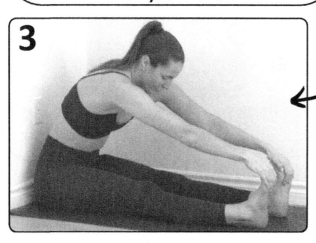

3

Hold this position, feeling a stretch in your hamstrings.

Side to Side Neck Rotations

BENEFITS

- Relieves tension and stiffness in the neck muscles.
- Increases neck mobility and flexibility.
- Promotes relaxation and can help reduce stress.

TIPS

- Keep your movements slow and controlled, focusing on the range of motion rather than speed. Allow your chin to lead the movement, ensuring a gentle rotation without straining.
- Breathe deeply and evenly throughout the exercise to enhance relaxation.
- Common Mistakes: Overextending or forcing the rotation can lead to strain. Keep the rotations within a comfortable range to prevent discomfort.

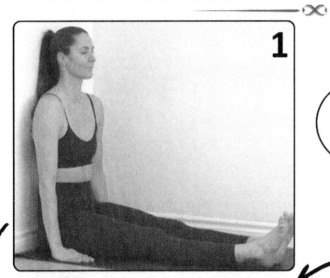

1

Start in a seated position with your back against the wall and your legs extended.

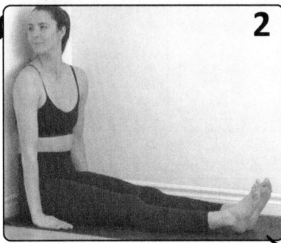

2

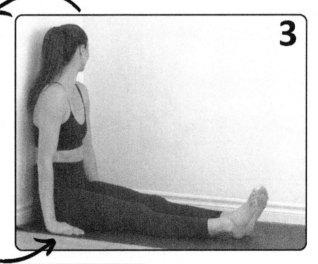

3

Gently rotate your neck from side to side, moving slowly from one side to the other.

Cat Cow

BENEFITS

- Enhances spinal flexibility and mobility.
- Relieves tension in the back and neck.
- Improves posture and body awareness.

TIPS

- As you push your hips back and round your spine (Cat Pose), focus on feeling a stretch along your spine.
- Flow smoothly between the two positions, synchronizing your movements with your breath for a calming effect.
- Breathe in as you extend into Cow Pose and exhale as you round into Cat Pose.
- Common Mistakes: Moving too quickly between positions can reduce the effectiveness of the stretches. Ensure each movement is deliberate and controlled.

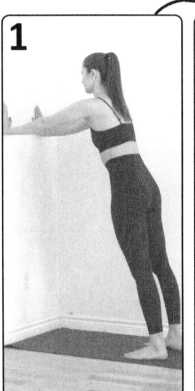

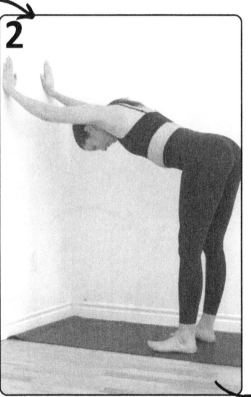

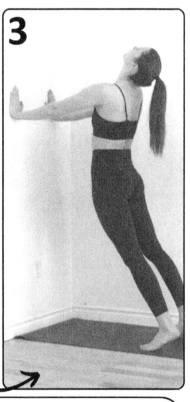

Stand facing the wall with your feet shoulder-width apart. Place your hands on the wall at chest level.

While keeping your hands in the same position, push your hips back to bring your chest towards the ground and round your spine. Hold briefly, then come back up, lift your chest as high as you can, looking up and extending your back. Continue this exercise by flowing through the two positions.

Butterfly Stretch

BENEFITS

- Opens and stretches the hips and inner thighs.
- Promotes flexibility in the lower body.
- Can help alleviate tightness and improve posture.

TIPS

- Sit with your back straight against the wall to support your spine.
- Bring the soles of your feet together, allowing your knees to fall to the sides. Gently press on your thighs with your hands or elbows for a deeper stretch, if comfortable.
- Focus on relaxing into the stretch rather than forcing your knees down.
- Breathe deeply and hold the stretch to allow your muscles to relax and open.
- Common Mistakes: Overpressing the knees or rounding the back can reduce the effectiveness of the stretch and potentially cause discomfort.

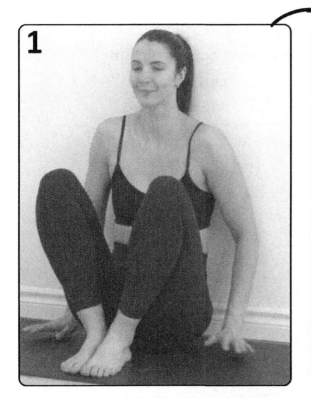

1 Start in a seated position with your back against the wall and your knees bent.

2 Bring the soles of your feet together and let your knees drop. Hold this position to open up the hips. You can also gently press down on your thighs for a deeper stretch.

Piriformis Stretch

BENEFITS

- Targets the piriformis muscle, reducing tightness and alleviating sciatic pain.
- Enhances hip flexibility and mobility.
- Can help improve lower back discomfort and posture.

TIPS

- Use your hand for slight pressure on the knee of the bent leg to deepen the stretch. Twist your torso gently towards the bent knee side to intensify the stretch without straining.
- Breathe deeply to allow the muscle to relax and stretch.
- Common Mistakes: Twisting too aggressively or applying too much pressure on the knee can strain the piriformis and hip joints. Keep the movement gentle and controlled.

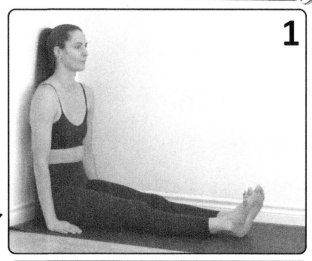

1

Start in a seated position with your back against the wall and your legs extended.

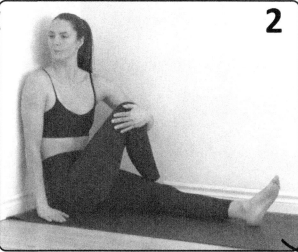

2

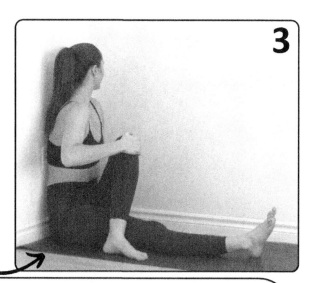

3

Bend your right knee and lift your foot, placing it on the outside of your left knee. Twist your upper body to the right to deepen the stretch (2). Repeat the exercise, switching the positions of your legs (3).

Single Leg Stretch

BENEFITS

- Enhances core strength and stability.
- Improves flexibility in the hips and hamstrings.
- Promotes coordination and control of leg movements.

TIPS

- Keep a slight bend in the knees to avoid over-straining the hamstrings.
- Lift your head and shoulders slightly to engage the core, maintaining a focused gaze towards your legs. Alternate legs smoothly, focusing on controlled movements and steady breathing.
- Common Mistakes: Jerking the leg towards the chest or lifting the lower back off the ground can compromise the effectiveness and safety of the stretch.

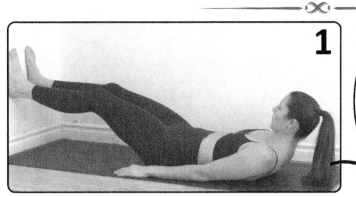

1 Lie on the ground on your back with your feet on the wall. Keep your legs straight with a gentle bend in your knees. Lift your head off the ground and hold this position.

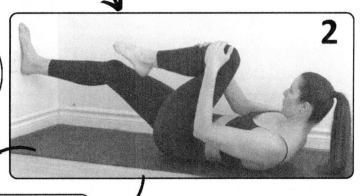

Bring one knee at a time towards your chest and use your arms to hug the leg in.

2

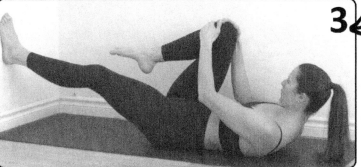

3 Hold briefly, then release the leg and repeat with the other leg. Continue by alternating legs each time.

Side Leg Swings

BENEFITS

- Increases hip mobility and lateral flexibility.
- Enhances muscle coordination and balance.
- Warms up the leg muscles, preparing them for exercise.

TIPS

- Start with gentle swings and gradually increase the range of motion as your muscles warm up.
- Keep the swinging leg straight, but not locked, to engage the muscles effectively.
- Focus on fluid, controlled movements rather than speed or force.
- Alternate legs to ensure balanced flexibility and mobility in both hips.
- Common Mistakes: Swinging the leg too forcefully from the start can lead to muscle strain. Maintain control throughout the movement to avoid injury.

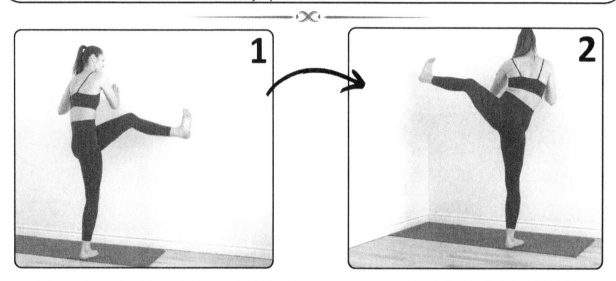

Stand with your feet hip-width apart facing a wall. Place both hands on the wall for support. Swing your left leg from your right side to your left side, using momentum to increase your range of motion.

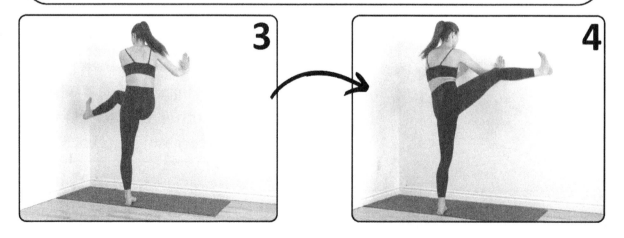

Wall Toe Touch Crunches

BENEFITS

- Targets the upper abdominals, enhancing core strength and definition.
- Promotes flexibility in the hamstrings.
- Engages the entire core for a comprehensive abdominal workout.

TIPS

- Keep your movements controlled, focusing on using your core to lift your shoulders off the ground. As you reach for your toes, aim to lift your upper back higher to deepen the crunch.
- Inhale as you prepare and exhale during the crunch to maximize core engagement.
- Common Mistakes: Jerking the neck or using momentum rather than controlled abdominal muscles can reduce effectiveness and increase the risk of injury.

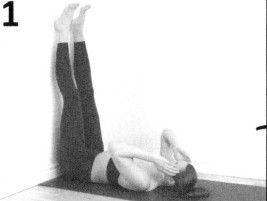

1

Lie on the ground with your legs up the wall. Keep your legs straight. Bend your elbows and place your hands by the sides of your head.

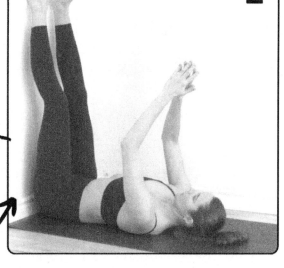

2

Contract your abdominals to lift your shoulder blades off the ground and reach for your toes

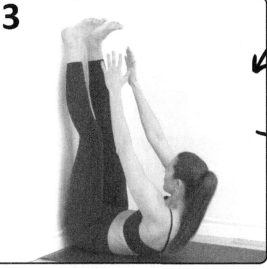

3

Slowly lower yourself back down and repeat.

Wall Supported Ankle Rolls

BENEFITS

- Improves ankle mobility and flexibility.
- Enhances circulation in the lower extremities.
- Can aid in preventing ankle injuries by strengthening the surrounding muscles.

TIPS

- Keep the standing leg slightly bent to engage the muscles and protect the knee. Roll the lifted ankle slowly, focusing on making complete and controlled circles.
- Perform equal numbers of rolls in both clockwise and counterclockwise directions to ensure balanced development. Alternate between the right and left ankle to promote equal mobility and strength.
- Common Mistakes: Rushing the ankle rolls or using too much pressure on the wall can reduce the effectiveness of the exercise. Ensure smooth, controlled movements for the best results.

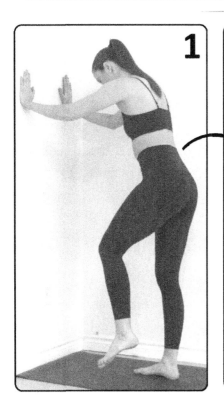

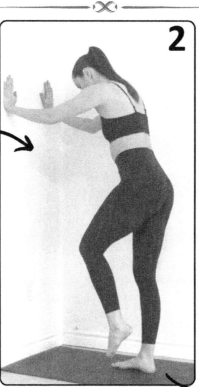

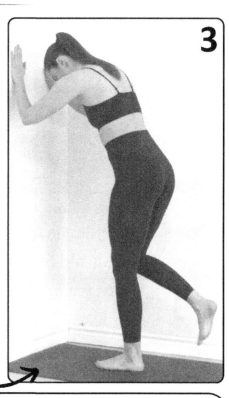

Stand facing a wall with your hands lightly resting on the wall for balance. Stand on your right foot, with a slight bend in the knee.

Lift your left foot off the ground, bending the knee slightly. Begin to roll your left ankle slowly, making circles with your toes. Perform the rolls in a clockwise direction,then switch the direction and roll your ankle counterclockwise. Repeat the exercise, switching the positions of your legs (3).

Keeping the Flame Alive: Overcoming Challenges and Staying Motivated

Embarking on a Wall Pilates journey is thrilling, but like any adventure, it comes with its ups and downs. This chapter is all about navigating those bumps in the road with grace and keeping the fire of motivation burning bright. Let's dive into overcoming these challenges together.

Addressing Common Physical and Emotional Barriers

Physical Hurdles: Sometimes, our bodies don't cooperate the way we want them to. Maybe it's tight hamstrings that make certain stretches feel impossible, or perhaps a lingering backache that's cramping your style. The key here is adaptation. Modify exercises to meet your body where it's at, using props like cushions for support or adjusting your stance to reduce strain. Remember, Wall Pilates is about celebrating what your body can do, not pushing it into submission.

Emotional Blocks: Then there are days when it's not your body but your mind putting up roadblocks. Maybe you're feeling too stressed, too tired, or just too blah to get moving. This is where small acts of self-compassion come in. Give yourself permission to have an off day, but also gently remind yourself why you started. Sometimes, just showing up is half the victory.

Tips for Consistency and Enjoyment

Find Your Why: Keeping your motivation high starts with having a clear, compelling reason for practicing Wall Pilates. Whether it's to gain strength, improve flexibility, or simply carve out some "me time," remind yourself of your why, especially on days when motivation is scarce.

Mix It Up: Routine is great, but variety is the spice of life – and of a sustainable Wall Pilates practice. Keep things fresh by introducing new exercises, challenging yourself with different sequences, or even changing up the time of day you practice. A little change can reignite your enthusiasm.

Tracking Progress and Celebrating Achievements

Set Milestones: Instead of focusing solely on the end goal, set smaller, achievable milestones along the way. Maybe it's mastering a challenging pose, noticing increased flexibility, or simply sticking with your practice for a full month. Recognizing these milestones gives you a sense of progress and accomplishment.

Keep a Pilates Journal: Documenting your Wall Pilates journey can be incredibly rewarding. Jot down exercises you've tried, how they felt, and any improvements you've noticed in your strength, flexibility, or mood. Over time, you'll have a tangible record of how far you've come.

Celebrate: Last but certainly not least, celebrate your achievements, no matter how small. Finished a week of workouts? Treat yourself to a relaxing bath. These celebrations keep the joy in your journey, fueling your motivation to keep going.

By embracing each part of your Wall Pilates journey, including its challenges, and celebrating every step, you create a rewarding and lasting practice. This holistic approach, supported by a balanced diet and complemented by practices like Yoga and mindfulness, enriches your overall well-being, crafting a fulfilling path to health that extends beyond the mat.

Workouts Index

The Final Stretch: Reflecting on Your Wall Pilates Journey

As we gently close the pages of our journey together through the transformative world of Wall Pilates, it's a moment to pause and reflect on the path we've navigated side by side. This book was conceived not merely as an instruction manual but as a companion on your journey to a deeper connection with your body and mind, using the simple yet profound support of a wall and the timeless wisdom of Pilates.

From the very first stretch to the concluding breath of our 28-Day Challenge, this guide aimed to illuminate the comprehensive benefits and adaptable nature of Wall Pilates. Beyond the intricacies of each movement and the tailored approaches for the unique phases of a woman's life, we delved into the symbiosis of physical exertion and mental clarity, hoping to bring you a practice that nurtures in totality.

As you step away from the wall and carry forward the lessons and strengths garnered, remember that every practice is a steppingstone to greater understanding and harmony within. Wall Pilates, with its foundation in mindfulness and physical well-being, is a testament to the continual journey of growth and self-discovery.

Thank you for embarking on this journey with me, for every stretch, breath, and moment of reflection shared. As we part ways, let's carry forward the essence of Wall Pilates into every aspect of our lives, embracing each new challenge with grace, strength, and the support of our ever-present wall.

With gratitude and warmth,

Thea Morrow

★★★★★

Hi! If you've found value in the workouts and guidance, I'd be incredibly grateful if you could take a moment to **leave a review.**

It's super **quick and easy**—just *scan the QR code to the left* with your cellphone to be taken directly to the review page.

Sharing your thoughts and experiences **takes less than 30 seconds** but **means a lot to me.**
Thank you for considering my request!

Printed in Great Britain
by Amazon

43370705R00066